DEPRESSION
THE COMEDY

Jessica Holmes

DEPRESSION
THE COMEDY

— A Tale of Perseverance —

PAGE TWO
BOOKS

Page Two Books
5 – 175 East 15th Avenue
Vancouver, B.C.
Canada V5T 2P6
www.pagetwobooks.com

Cataloguing data available from Library and Archives Canada
ISBN 978-0-9952665-4-4 (paperback)
ISBN 978-1-989025-14-7 (ebook)

Produced by Page Two Books
Cover design by Peter Cocking and Michelle Clement
Cover illustration by Michelle Clement
Cover photo by Rodney Daw Photography
Interior design by Peter Cocking
Interior illustrations by Jessica Holmes
Interior photos courtesy Jessica Holmes
Photos on p. 22 and p. 75 by iStockphoto
Printed and bound in Canada by Friesens
www.jessicaholmes.com

For Pat.

Contents

1   Hi There, [Insert Your Name Here]................ 1

2   Everything Is Funny... Eventually................ 9

3   I Got This Oprah Gig............................... 27

4   Miss Piggy.. 41

5   Marriage Is So Fun for the First
    Couple of Years! 51

6   It Takes a Village to Save a Marriage........... 77

7   Humiliation Fee 99

8   Invent the Invisibility Cloak Already! 113

9   The Kids Are the Boss of Me.....................129

10   What Comes First: The Comedian
     or the Depression?...................................147

11   So Here's the Thing................................ 171

    Acknowledgments......................................187

    Some Resources 189

Hi There,
[Insert Your Name Here]

* * * * *

HI THERE, [insert your name here]. So glad you've got the energy to pick up a book. You're miles ahead of the old me already! I'm assuming you're here for one of the following reasons:

- You've experienced depression somewhere on a scale of a little "I get sad every January" to a lot "my psychiatrist doesn't have a name for what I've got."
- Your employer gave you this book to create a culture of compassion so you won't be awkward next time "Anxious Jody" gets back from stress leave.
- You think comedians, especially the unstable ones, are a barrel of monkeys (we are!).

Whatever the case: welcome. Take off your socks and make yourself comfortable!

Laughter may seem like an odd approach to a book about sadness. But there are already thousands of determinedly serious books on the subject, and thousands more self-help books about healing your own noggin through mindfulness and gritty smoothies that I'm sure would do us all a world of good (ya know, if you had the energy, time, inclination...). Personally I've bought dozens of them and usually only made it through the first chapter. Now if they just made one big book with only first chapters of other books, THAT I could get through! Anyway, this un-serious, un-helpful book is meant merely as a reminder that no one is alone in their problems, and that, eventually, if you let a whopping amount of time pass, you might find a kernel of levity in the muck. Humour is one heck of a coping mechanism, am I right, [insert your name here]? Actually, [insert your name here], inserting your name everywhere is gonna make this more like a passport renewal application than a casual chat, so let's give you a name. Are you more of a Jacob or a Jennifer? Or something millennial-ish like Riley? Let's just call you Pat. Am I right, Pat?

PAT: Uh, yes.
ME: Great. You're doing great.

Well, Pat, since we're on a first-name basis, I might as well admit that (*exaggerated sigh*) what you're reading is actually The Introduction. I didn't want to label it as such because introductions usually seem dry, like they were written by someone wearing a monocle. Or worse, two monocles! Feel free to *not* read it—when you turn eighteen you can live by your own rules and eat pizza for breakfast and skip introductions. But in this case I do have pertinent information I want to get across before we dive right in. That ok?

PAT: Sure. I assumed this was the introduction. It has "Hi There" in the title.

ME: Oh. Right. Well, in that case I'm very impressed that you didn't skip over it. You probably eat salads with every meal and paid attention to supply teachers as a child, am I right?

PAT: Well, not r—

ME: Sorry, Pat, but I've gotta move things along. Where was I? Ah yes, depression!

So, since depression is a mental illness, and not an obviously physical one like chicken pox or scurvy, it's difficult to quantify. But these are some guidelines that help us describe it slightly more specifically than "Sally's a total b!#&h lately!"

By the Mayo Clinic's definition, depression is experiencing at least five of the following symptoms most of the day, nearly every day. I've put them in a loosey-goosey font so they're not such a downer. And I've added a * next to the ones I experienced. Fun game! Play along if you like.

- Feelings of sadness, emptiness, or unhappiness*

- Angry outbursts, irritability, or frustration, even over small matters*

- Loss of interest or pleasure in normal activities, such as sex*

- Sleep disturbances, including insomnia or sleeping too much*

- Tiredness and lack of energy, so that even small tasks take extra effort*

- Changes in appetite—often reduced appetite and weight loss

- Anxiety, agitation, or restlessness*
- Slowed thinking, speaking, or body movements*
- Feelings of worthlessness or guilt*
- Trouble thinking, concentrating, making decisions, and remembering*
- Frequent thoughts of death, suicidal thoughts, suicide attempts, or suicide (if you're experiencing anything even close to this one, skip right to the resource list at the back of the book!)
- Unexplained physical problems, such as back pain or headaches

If you have five or more of these symptoms, Dr. Mayo's website says you may be depressed. If you have fewer than a handful but more than none, then you may be in what Dr. Seuss calls a slump—which also feels terrible, but doesn't qualify you for certain health care benefits. Either way, read on!

A bit about me: I'd make a terrible detective. Like, just the worst. Despite ALL the clues, I didn't realize I was depressed until I'd spent two years in the gutter. And I'm a professional comedian, which I assumed would have made it easier to detect, 'cause going from the life of the party to a downer seems like a more obvious transition than going from, say, a mortician to a downer. But maybe I just don't know morticians like I think I do.

Like anyone who's been down, I asked: Why me? My only weak spot growing up had been over-sensitivity. Like bawling when the dog ate my homemade zucchini-head doll or when my mom got upset instead of laughing after my brother and I painted a toilet paper roll brown and put it back in the dispenser—"What the heck is wrong with you deviants?!"—as though she had never even heard of prop comedy. But I always bounced back, excited to see what else the day held, whether writing funny stories, breeding finches, or acting out scenes from the *Airplane!* movies:

"Surely you can't be serious!"
"I am serious. And don't call me Shirley!"

Classic!

So there I was at the start of 2012: my kids were carefree; my husband was a tall, supportive actor with thick hair who loved doing dishes; and my career was a strange adventure (one day I'm pitching a sitcom, the next I'm advertising chicken, the next I'm performing stand-up comedy for kids, pretending I can't hear the smart*ss eight-year-old in the front row who keeps saying, "I just don't get her"). I played basketball, belonged to a great group of friends, and loved my mom and dad. This modern-day Camelot lifestyle is where my depression started. This is where something malfunctioned.

Slipping from

"Woo-hoo!"

to a funk

to a depression

happened so gradually that it went unnoticed. Having already experienced postpartum depression years earlier, I figured I'd know the warning signs: anxiously crying and thinking, "I can't look after my kids because I love them so much that it paralyzes me with fear." But therapy and the right drugs helped me through that awful four-month episode and I had been going about life freely, thinking, "Phew, glad that's done with!" as though it was a suspicious mole I'd had removed. I would never experience that crippling fear for my kids' safety again (just the usual helicopter-parent fear that they'll be sneezed on, be bullied by a fellow toddler, or play with a toy from China that has lead in the paint). This depression was different. It snuck up on me without cause, disguised as many other things.

Over the course of a year I moved from a 9 out of 10 on the scale of life satisfaction, to feeling like waking up every morning was punishment. I resented fun stuff like girls' night out, developed a loathing for words like "wellness," hid from my agents, and avoided foods that promised to prolong my life. Even yawning through an emceeing gig for Oprah—despite the fact that she had long been a hero of mine—didn't sound any alarms for me. Years into this sludge, when my husband finally dragged me to see a marriage counsellor who declared me depressed in our second meeting, I realized I'd gone from cheerleader to zombie without ever noticing. See, Pat, I'd make a terrible detective! My friend Anson should have detected it much sooner; he's so dedicated to '80s crime sleuths that when he visited the *Magnum, P.I.* set on his honeymoon in Hawaii, he wore nothing but a pair of red Tom Selleck short-shorts. I'm sure I've got a picture of that here somewhere—

PAT: Uh, Jess?
ME: Yes?

PAT: Are you done with the introduction?
ME: Yes, actually.

A few notes in closing:

- This book is a collection of chapters—some on point (I Got This Oprah Gig), some batty (Miss Piggy)—about different areas of my life that were impacted by depression.
- It's my screwball take on my personal experience, not reflective of depressions in general, so take it with a grain of salt, or a dill pickle or something.
- It will be more impactful if you imagine it being read by Morgan Freeman. So... do that.

Happy reading! (Or unhappy reading. I really don't want to pressure you.)

Everything Is Funny...
Eventually

* * * * *

ME: PAT! CONGRATS on making it past the introduction! I consider this a success. Probably because I abandon a lot of books a few pages in. I also leave a lot of movies a few minutes in. I mean, if the popcorn's gone by the end of the previews, why bother hanging around? But you're here! You've doven right in! Wait, that doesn't sound right. Is "doven" a word?

PAT: No.

ME: Disregard it then. It's not pivotal to the story. In fact *none* of my stories are pivotal to the story. We're just here for fun. And that's what this chapter's about: fun. Now imagine I made some poignant segue and dig in!

Comedy writers live by the mantra that

Tragedy + Time = Comedy

and that the best comedy comes from real life. I knew this on a gut level when I was a kid. Any time something odd or uncomfortable happened, I'd process it as my own personalized sitcom. My fodder was usually based on family events. I jotted down the details when my far-sighted great aunt sat down and talked to a life-sized stuffed Santa doll for twenty minutes without realizing it wasn't human; when my dad swerved to miss hitting an ample lady in a blue muumuu dawdling across the road, then said, "Phew, if we had hit her, there'd be blueberry jam everywhere"; when my young cousins begged their parents to visit the ocean, but my aunt and uncle didn't have the money to take them across the country, so they just drove their kids an hour to Lake Ontario and said: "This is the Atlantic Ocean. Isn't it majestic?!"

Hanging out with my family was like being in a sitcom. We were all clearly defined characters: My mom, Laura, was an agnostic feminist social worker who was perpetually volunteering or taking night classes. My dad, Randy, was, and I can't think of a different way of putting this, a zany Mormon computer engineer. Also, he cooked weirdly. Not badly. Just weirdly— spaghetti and giblets, macaroni and hoof. You get the gist.

PAT: I don't. I don't get the gist.
ME: Then consider yourself lucky.

Despite being fraternal twins, my brother Marcus was an athlete with a hundred friends and my brother George was an introvert who skewered Hollywood A-listers for fun. And me, I was a sensitive, gangly kid with the attention span of a goldfish who took up a new hobby every couple of months. My parents were relieved when my "making dolls out of old zucchinis" phase was replaced by sewing cat clothing. (The cat was relieved when that phase was replaced by scratch-and-sniff sticker collecting.)

This was a fairly standard dinner conversation:

RANDY: (*wrapping up a prayer*)... and please bless this cow tongue stroganoff, that it may make us strong. In the name of Jesus Christ, amen.

MARCUS: Amen.

LAURA: Thank the Goddess!

ME: Is God a lady?

RANDY: No.

LAURA: Prove it!

GEORGE: I pray to the big box office in the sky that Tom Hanks will become a real actor, and not an overpaid, puppy-eyed lackey.

RANDY: Eat up, George.

GEORGE: Uh, thank you, good sir, but I must decline. I'm not the biggest fan of cow tongue. It's like we're kissing with each bite.

LAURA: Well, now I don't want mine, either.

MARCUS: Heads-up—I reserve the phone tonight.

(*SILENCE*)

ME: What do you mean? Like, *all* night?

MARCUS: Yeah, I have some friends calling about a game.

ME: From now till like, 10 p.m.? That's four hours!

MARCUS: What do *you* need the phone for? You gonna call the cat or something?

RANDY: Jess, you can play Donkey Kong with me. Let's make it a tournament.

ME: But I have so much homework.

RANDY: Yeah, but you can always skip that.

LAURA: (*head in hands*) Goddess, give me strength!

Out came a scrap of paper, an old receipt, a gum wrapper, and I'd scribble 'er down.

I'd cut out newspaper headlines that struck me as funny, like "Man Grateful for First Seeing Eye Pony" (some folks in Raleigh decided Seeing Eye dogs were for losers and invented/bred/trained the first Seeing Eye pony. It took them a while to work out the kinks, including trying to get the pony to not sneak chocolate bars on its trial run to the grocery store). And "Science Teacher Scolded for Telling Children Santa Would Burst into Flames" (if he really travelled fast enough to visit every child's house in one night).

My scraps weren't jokes. Just scenes or moments I wanted to hang on to, because they were compelling, or funny, or ridiculous, like when I discovered there's such a thing as the Housekeeping Olympics, where the winningest hotel room cleaning staff takes home the Golden Toilet Brush award.

What a wonderful world.

I collected these tidbits the way you might PVR your favourite TV shows. They were the closest I ever came to having imaginary friends. I've heard this from other introverts—your imagination is like its own person. You're "hanging out together" when you're alone. I mean, I never went as far as hugging myself and humming "Just the Two of Us," but I was content. And being on my own always seemed easier anyway, given I'm terrified of even the slightest confrontation.

PAT: Really? You get on a stage in front of strangers for a living, but you're afraid of confrontation?

ME: Yeah. Like, even on my very first date, when a bird dropping landed on my date's spiky mohawk, I didn't tell him because I was uncomfortable delivering bad news. We sat through the entirety of *Gremlins 2: The New Batch* while I guiltily avoided looking at him and the white-ish blob suspended an inch above his head.

PAT: That's beyond being scared of confrontation. That's verging on rude.

ME: Potatoes, patatoes.

When I was on a roll with an idea, it would trump my social life—even as a teen.

FRIEND: Let's go to the mall to celebrate your birthday. I'll shoplift you a present!

ME: I can't. My dad just passed a kidney stone, and he's put it in a decorative jar that he wants to display on the mantle, and my mom's going nuts. I wanna turn it into a scene.

FRIEND: A scene for what? A movie?

ME: No, just, for... putting on paper.

Maybe that's why I had just a few close friends but never kept up with acquaintances; you take a rain check so you can doodle one too many times and people move on.

I hung up and lay back on the bed, lingering in my imagination, picturing how the kidney stone scenario would play out the funniest. Then I jotted the scene down on a piece of paper I'd inevitably lose track of, but I'd still get some odd comfort from it being recorded.

Being scribble-worthy became a bit of a contest within my family, and my grandparents put up a list on their fridge to keep track of who was worth quoting, or not.

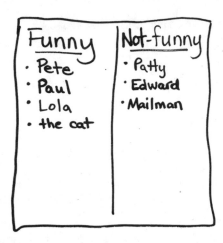

Soon enough, in the middle of conversations, people would turn and ask, "Aren't you going to write that down?" and I'd mime writing something so no feelings got hurt. I wasn't waiting to be *told* something funny (and definitely wasn't waiting for people to re-enact jokes they heard on TV), I was waiting to be surprised by people being their colourful, unpredictable selves.

When my mom replaced a hot dog with a bulrush and served it to my uncle as a protest against men expecting women to serve them, I scribbled. When I was learning to drive and my dad advised me to "really put the pedal to the metal when you're going over a hill so you feel it in your stomach" or when my grandmother brought out a cake on Christmas and made us sing "Happy Birthday" to baby Jesus, I scribbled. And when my grandfather confided he'd been poor as a child "so there were a lot of IOUs from the tooth fairy," well, I hugged him, then I scribbled.

I'm very close with my grandparents. My grandfather, who spent most of his career helping Vietnamese immigrants settle in to life in the town of Peterborough, patiently taught me to cook (which I'm just realizing now was his gentle way of giving me an alternative to the weird meats and gelatins my father was always cooking up). He had a tin of cue-card recipes for rolled sandwiches, chicken pot pie, gravy—his gravy was so good that he'd make extra so he could send fans home with a jar (this was long before "cholesterol" was a household word). We made butter tarts from scratch. I rolled out the crust, and loved the satisfaction of putting each cut-out piece into the muffin pan in a perfect little nest for the butter and sugar filling. Mmmm butter and sugar filling...

PAT: Jess!
ME: Yes?
PAT: Uh, you trailed off there.
ME: Whoops. Sorry! Just fantasizing about having teenage metabolism again.

Anyway, when I mentioned to my grampa that my friend Tara and I were going backpacking through Europe after high school, he offered to join us on the last leg of the trip. Though Tara wasn't convinced that bringing senior citizens to Europe was what the cool kids were doing, I was elated. His presence would solidify my philosophy that the world is my sitcom.

One night he and I were walking down an unusually empty street in Paris, and a sports car pulled up. The driver, a snazzy man in a flashy silver suit, started barking rapid-fire instructions at us. I couldn't place his accent, but understood enough of his broken English to decipher, "I'm lost and need directions. Come close to the car. Give me your wallets. I'm not robbing you. Exchange only. Special packages for you!"

Huh?

ME: Oh gosh. Thanks, but we're not interested.

He wouldn't let up. He was aggressively schmoozy, like one of those perfume-sample guys at the mall who traps you into engaging by asking, "Has anyone ever told you you've got a beautiful smile?" and you kind of feel like not answering would be admitting that "no, no one ever tells me that," but replying gives him the green light to badger you with forceful flattery until you buy an eighty dollar jar of toilet water (everything sounds better in French!), because of course we wouldn't hand over our money. I mean, seriously,

a. he wasn't armed, and
b. we were doing Europe on $5 a day, as I was saving up for university. We'd been eating mainly day-old bread and processed cheese, washing our clothes in the sink, and sleeping in sixteen-people-per-room hostels to cut costs. Every dollar I had was precious.

But this hustler kept calling, "Come closer! Wallets! Not robbery! I give you jackets!" and maybe because Grampa was a pious man who had never cared for material things, or because he'd been playing fast and loose ever since joining a seniors' song-and-dance troupe the year before, or because Canadians are just that nice... he pulled his wallet out of his fanny pack and shrugged, "Well, I'll bite." The man snatched it. And perhaps because I was suffering from Stockholm Syndrome after only two minutes, or because I didn't want to appear like I didn't trust Grampa's wisdom, I handed over my wallet, too. The fancy grifter took out the money, tossed back our empty wallets, and threw two packages at our feet, then sped away calling, "I have not robbed youuuuuuuuuu." I watched him leave in disbelief. If it weren't for the packages on the sidewalk, I'd have wondered if the whole hurried exchange was a figment of my imagination. I tore open the packages, hoping the jackets he spoke of were worth the hundreds of dollars he'd taken. I pulled out two teeny, pleather, Michael Jackson–style coats.

What the...

They were small. Like, little. They'd barely have fit a Cabbage Patch doll.

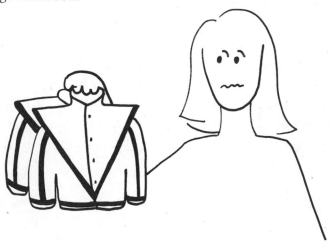

Dang it, he did rob us!

I heard my grampa wheezing behind me.

Plus, Grampa's having a stroke!

I turned to see him bent over at the waist, laughing. Laughing. So. Darn. Hard.

ME: Grampa, what are you laughing about?! We just gave away all our money, and all we have to show for it are these stupid, miniature jackets!

He looked at the tiny jackets and laughed even harder. I sat on the curb and watched him, shaking my head. After a minute, his laughter died down and he looked me in the eye with a sympathetic smile.

GRAMPA: Jess, we weren't paying for the jackets. We were paying for the story.

Huh.

I'd eat a bucket of gravy with him, anytime.

When, after my first year of university, I travelled to Venezuela as a missionary (I had followed in my father's footsteps and joined the Mormon church a year earlier), I purchased a notebook to serve as my first official Funny Journal so that my ideas were recorded like this:

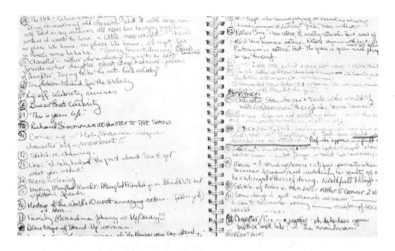

And no longer like this:

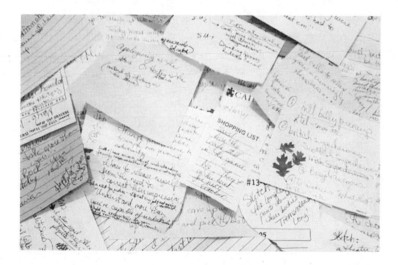

I'd lie down in my single bed at night, with a "Sister" (the title given to our missionary companion) across from me listening to any number of pre-approved Christian tracks on her

Sony Walkman, and take a break from scratching my mosquito bites to jot down the day's highlights:

- local kids chasing us with a bucket of pee, to punish our non-Catholicness, I presume
- trying to teach a lady about the church, but she spent the whole hour distractingly snuggling her lap-chicken
- hiding Sister So-and-so's used socks in her pillowcase and waiting to see if she sensed anything out of the ordinary when she went to bed. She did not, and just thought we were idiots when we tattled on ourselves (but since she's not allowed to use the word "idiots," she insultingly declared, "You're so silly," which only made us laugh harder)

When I made the difficult decision to leave the Mormon church a few years later, in part because their whole "don't be all homosexual" thing didn't jive with my values, I made another journal entry.

- I called my mother, crying: "But what if I don't get into Mormon heaven?" She sighed and said, "Then it'll be you, me, and the gays in limbo." That made me feel better, and is also, for all I know, accurate. It would make for one heck of a party, though!

Once I started getting offers to write and perform on comedy series, I gathered my many years of journals and scraps and they became my muse. Quirks and characters that had lived in my imagination for twenty-five years poured out. But turning your creative hobby, your happy-maker, into your *job* has its pitfalls, particularly if that hobby is the cornerstone of your personality. I dove in heart-first and got attached to the thrill and the joy and the frou-frou of television so quickly, like a girl who starts planning her wedding on the first date. When the first series I worked on wasn't renewed after a single season, I figured "easy come, easy go," and hoped I'd land somewhere just as marvellous real soon. When the second series also wasn't renewed past one season, I thought, "Wow, all those characters, done. Oh well, onward and upward!" Third series, exact same fate. But I brushed myself off, knowing the phrase "First World problems" was written for soft disappointments like this. A year later I was offered my own Carol Burnett-style series, and it was a dream come true. My friends and I wrote and performed sketches, songs, and impressions, letting our inner dorks shine with complete childlike playfulness. Creativity flowed through me, and it was a lifetime high.

YES! This is it!!

I'm home.

But then... it happened again. Terminated. This time, several of the writers and performers from my series were offered work on a new, similar comedy project, minus me. And much like the plot of the '60s pop song "It's My Party and I'll Cry If I Want To," I felt like my boyfriend had dumped me for my best friend. Yes, this type of thing happens all the time in entertainment, and sure, in clichéd terms I still had my health, and maybe, as I often told myself, "No one is owed anything in this business. Get over it already!" But reasonably or not, it broke my spirit a little... well, maybe even a lot.

If this was my very best, and I gave it everything I had,

and it STILL got cancelled,

what's the point?

I must have made the unconscious decision that I would not reach for the highs to avoid the risk of hitting the lows, because I stopped pitching TV series.

And I stopped scribbling down funny ideas.

Jeepers, what a bummer. Here's a stock photo of a kitten to get us back on track:

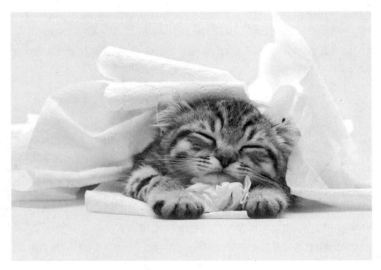

After a very dry year and a half of temping to pay the bills, and moving in with my boyfriend Scott because I loved him (and also because it cut those bills in half), I was thrilled and surprised and relieved to be hired on the well-established comedy series *Royal Canadian Air Farce*. The show had been running a steady fifteen seasons already, so the chance of it being cancelled the moment I stepped on board would be, to borrow a term from that guy in *Princess Bride*, "incontheivable."

I've landed! I've landed!

Two of the greatest mentors I could ask for, Roger Abbott and Don Ferguson, welcomed me aboard and the show fit me like a warm mitten. Their writers had me playing Michael Jackson (it felt surprisingly natural to see him as a white woman), Britney Spears (it was during her shaved-head phase, and, I have to say, bald is not a great look on me), and Céline Dion (pro wrestler Trish Stratus was a guest star and we shot a fight scene where she twirled me over her head and threw me out a window). What's not to love?

Still, I couldn't shake my writer's block.

Anything I put on paper came from a scarcity mindset, like I was in a pressure cooker—"When am I gonna get my next hit of funny? Mama has bills to pay!" Lacking my usual sense of playful improvisation, when I did stand-up, I'd stick to variations of the same jokes I'd written years earlier.

So this is what a hack feels like? Huh. Could be worse.

I had stopped being a spectator, and losing that invisible friend had more of an impact than I realized.

It was only years later, when I had gone through and recovered from depression, that I felt a desire to start jotting down funnies again. That's the only silver lining I can think of for depression—the brand new re-appreciation of life when you finally come out of the dark and feel genuine laughter as if for the first time, and you think, "Oh, this feels so much better than I ever remember it! I'm really gonna appreciate the good times."

PAT: And empathy.

ME: Pardon me?

PAT: You probably have more empathy for other people, now.

ME: Well, aren't you the keener! (*pause*) Yes, actually, when I recovered I had more empathy, too. So laughter and empathy are the pots of gold at the end of the turd rainbow that is depression.

PAT: You should make bumper stickers for a living.

ME: I think you meant that sarcastically, but I'm gonna take it as a compliment!

A few months after I was diagnosed, and dutifully seeking treatment, some relatives were visiting with their dog, Gracie, a small, golden-ish poodle mix whose breed I haven't memorized on principle because there are just too many variations now and if I can't remember my passwords half the time, then I'm sure not going to bother trying to keep up with expensive dog breeds. Anyway, our cheap mutt, Ellie, who we had recently adopted on the advice of my new psychiatrist "so you'll be forced to leave the house," had a little yellow stuffed dog toy that looked like Gracie. At one point, Gracie went behind the kitchen island, and Scott (by now my husband— way to go, Jess!), also behind the island, kicked the stuffed toy across the room and shouted, "Gracie, are you ok?"

In his defence, there were only about two seconds when we thought that he had kicked the real dog, and he was very good-natured about the angry eye rolls he got. I didn't laugh out loud at another one of his questionable "jokes," but I did smile. When our relatives left, I went down to the basement

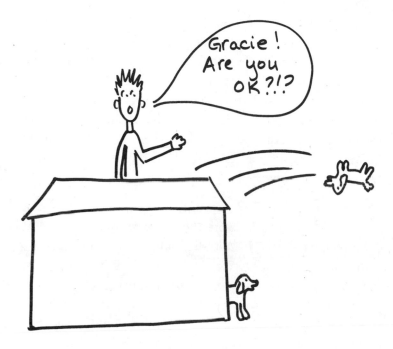

office, and combed through a cabinet of old wrapping paper, stationery, odd socks, and found it: my funny journal. I added the evening's shenanigans, and brought it upstairs to show Scott. We combed through some of the entries and found one of my favourites:

- Scott's hairdresser had a large, uncovered wart on his finger and kept running his fingers through Scott's hair. When Scott asked him to put a bandage over the wart, the hairdresser said, "But it's not contagious. It just transfers from one person's skin to another."

ME: That was a good one.
SCOTT: Heh-heh. Yeah. Gross.

My funny journal isn't for profit. I'm not recording these events to turn them into jokes someday. They're just for... joy. For mental health. At the very least, they remind me that life is usually more comedy than tragedy, and at their not-least (is that how you say that?), they reaffirm the lesson my grandfather taught me: our experiences, even the oddball ones, create a tapestry of memories that tie us together. They're my comedy quilt!

My most recent funny journal is just a memo app on my phone. My latest entry is:

- I was invited to give a keynote speech on depression in Ottawa, but a week before the presentation I realized my speech would be given in the middle of a mall, like I was a contestant on *Star Search: The Sad Version*. I called my dad to get emotional support for what would clearly be an embarrassing event where I pour out my soul to an audience of shoppers who stop to listen for all of five seconds. When he heard I'd be speaking at a mall, he exclaimed, "Jess, you're as important as Santa!"

Some failures become punchlines, and that reminds me that mistakes are ok. My funny journal frames life as a win-win for me: when things are good, they're good, and when they're bad, I'll probably laugh about them eventually anyway. And I'm noticing lately, when I mark these ideas down, I get a familiar feeling of "welcome back, friend."

I Got This Oprah Gig

. . . . .

ME: HEY, PAT. You're just in time for me to explain the difference between a funk and a depression—hope you brought popcorn!

Ahem. Long ago, the guy who purchased Louisiana said, "With great r—"

PAT: Thomas Jefferson? He arranged the Louisiana Purchase. He didn't *buy* Louisiana.
ME: Well, thanks for keeping me honest, Pat.

Nevertheless, the guy who did that thing once said, "With great risk comes great reward." And that's the motto ambitious comedians live by. In my twenties I soaked up every motivational philosophy I could get from Oprah

"You become what you believe"

to Herman Melville

"It is better to fail in originality than to succeed in imitation"

27

to Blake from *Glengarry Glen Ross*

"Always be closing."

I felt like there was an answer (or at least a cliché) for every problem, and I could only succeed or fail by my own chutzpa. And ya know something, Pat? It worked. For all the embarrassing times I had to pay my dues by wearing a mascot costume, doing poolside comedy, or impersonating Martha Stewart while handing out stinky cheese to partygoers who were completely embarrassed for me, I'm happy to say, it all paid off! Unfortunately, the payoff came smack in the middle of my undiagnosed depression, so I've basically experienced great success and been extremely sad about it. That's the state I was in when my hero came to town...

ME: *Doodly-doodly-doodly-doodly-d—*
PAT: What are you doing?
ME: Making flashback sound effects.
PAT: Wow.
ME: I know, right?!

INT. HOUSE. DAY.
We pan down the stairs to a cluttered basement rec room. At the far corner is a blue sectional. On it lies Jessica, late thirties, in a unitard painted to look like a business suit (think full-body tuxedo shirt). She is surrounded by empty calorie-reduced pudding cups and cracker boxes. The clock reads 2:36 p.m. Jessica coughs lightly in her sleep. She wakes and checks her phone.

In the spring of 2012, my BlackBerry bleeped with the happy news that THE Oprah Winfrey was blessing Toronto with a visit. I rose from the comfort and safety of my blue sofa, stretched out the kinks, and walked to the next room, where my computer sat in its forty-eighth hour of rest mode.

This would be so much easier if I had one
of those old-people scooters.

I took the cat off the keyboard, nodded up at Oprah on my vision board, and ordered a pair of tickets for her one-day-only show. "Oprah can turn our luck around," I told the cat, who pretended not to hear me. Back to the sofa I went, proud of having done a thing.

Less than twenty-four hours after the irresponsible purchase, I got a call from a producer I've worked with asking if I'd emcee the event.

ME: Just a sec, I gotta sit up for this.
PRODUCER: Huh?
ME: This is a big deal. Really. Thanks. (*sigh*) But shoot. I already bought tickets. Can I get a refund?
PRODUCER: No.
ME: Oh well. I'd love to emcee regardless. Neat.

Neat?

A major coup for my bucket list and all I could think was "neat"? Neat is a 30% OFF promo code for GAP. Neat is finding jeans under the bed that smell clean enough you wear them a third day in a row.

ME: Something doesn't add up here, cat.
CAT: (*silence*)

I sat with the news for a few minutes, waiting for the moment when it would feel real, when I would believe it. A therapist later told me that depressed minds are like a sieve that only allows negative information to pass through.

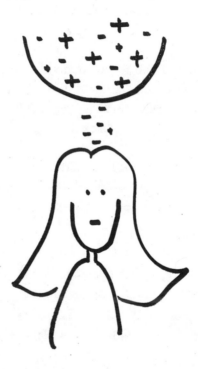

My brain's little sieve continued to accept neat, and some doubt. But not a single trace of

*E*P*I*C*

Twenty minutes later, when I couldn't push past feeling doubtfully neat I decided to ignore the news. I didn't call my agents, who would have drummed me up a mountain of publicity:

"MEDIUM-TOWN GIRL OPENS FOR GREATEST HUMAN"

Nor did I drop the standard humblebrag online: "omg Oprah must have terrible taste cause I'm one of her 'Favourite Things' lol #blessed #lucky #annoying." Didn't start writing customized jokes, or visualize receiving a standing ovation so grand that a defeated Oprah, standing backstage, shrugs and says to Gayle, "No point trying to go on after that." Instead, still splayed out on the sofa with *Dr. Phil* on pause, I made a whiny mental list of all the gigs that had been promised to me but had never materialized. It's kind of a given in the entertainment industry that things fall through. It happens at the A-list level ("They just booted Terrence Howard out of the next *Iron Man*") and at my humble Canadian level ("Things fell through and you won't be the next Stephanie Massicotte") (she's a weather girl in Saskatoon). I even had a sold-out show opening for one of my idols cancelled the night before due to a contractual dispute between the idol and the producer. (Maybe not enough rose-scented candles or green M&M's? I never found out anything beyond "these things happen.") Insecurity is such a given that most actors learn not to get invested until they're actually on set, just to make sure they don't yell, "Smell you later, a#&hole" at the manager of the restaurant where they're waiting tables until they know the starring role was a sure thing. But there's a difference between not counting your chickens before they hatch and telling eager, available chickens to f#$k off. I knew I'd been in a funk lately (by lately, I mean a few years), but I assumed my personal lack of fanfare was either me needing more iron in my diet or having off-the-charts humility.

I guess I'm so grounded that giant career coups slide off my back!

Intimidated by the pressure to make the most of this rare and exciting opportunity, I thought it wisest to tuck into a ball and go back to watching *Dr. Phil* chastise deviants.

Peace.

When Scott got home I shared the great news.

ME: Hey, you can give one of those Oprah tickets I bought to a friend, 'cause I might be working the show.
SCOTT: What do you mean? You're gonna be onstage with her?
ME: I dunno. Someone called and asked if I'd emcee. But who knows.
SCOTT: Wow! That's amaz—
ME: Hon, can you keep it down, please. I just want some peace and quiet while I finish off this box of cheese-flavoured crackers.
SCOTT: Oh, ok. Did you have a... tough day?
ME: Well, it was busy, 'cause I unloaded half the dishwasher this morning, then there was that Oprah call this aft, so now I just need to relax with the TV and de-stress.
SCOTT: Oh. Ok. Well, congratulat—
ME: Scott, shhhhh PLEASE!!!

He skulked out of the room and I winced into my pillow.

I bet Robin never snaps at Dr. Phil like that.

I switched the channel to *America's Next Top Model*, hoping—

Pat: Whoa! Wait, your husband was there?

ME: Yeah.

PAT: Well, didn't he notice how much time you spent on the sofa every day?

ME: Huh. I guess in retrospect it's pretty weird that he didn't say anything about it. Maybe my bar had lowered so gradually that neither one of us reached an "aha moment," to quote my new buddy, Oprah. Like the stories of doomed frogs who don't jump out of a pot of water on the stove because they don't recognize the change in temperature from cold to boiling if it's gradual enough. But now that I think about it, we were kinda clueless.

PAT: That's more than clueless. That's, like, stu—

ME: Whoa, ha-ha. Hey! I'm sort of in a groove with the story right now, and I've got whole chapters on Scott, so, I'm just gonna keep on truckin'.

Months passed. I had a gig here and there, and otherwise spent my days lamenting how the grass is always greener anywhere but here. "I bet the people who work at banks aren't sobbing about failed potential and eating ice cream out of the bucket with a fork they dug out from the sofa cushions right now." A nagging buzz kept telling me to seize the day and splash my news across the internet, but the stronger that feeling got, the more I clung to my sectional for dear life and turned up the volume on reality shows to distract me. I knew something wasn't right, but sort of the same way you don't pick at the corners of trippy '70s wallpaper because there may be even trippier '60s wallpaper underneath, I felt like if I just kept pressing ahead, I could out-ignore the abyss forming beneath me.

I just have to keep my mind occupied.

Watching Tyra Banks tell a girl that she had to smile less with her mouth and more with her eyes while I practised along at home made me feel like I was doing something.

I have goals!

Scott texted from upstairs, "Are you picking up the kids from school today?" and I texted back, "No, I'm so busy."
I hadn't been to the schoolyard in months. Too many people.

PEOPLE: So what are you up to lately? Scott says you're opening for Oprah?
ME: It's probably not going to happen.
PEOPLE: Oh. Still. Oprah, I mean, I'd love to be in your shoes.

And then I'd smile (with mouth *and* eyes) as a sign I was humbly accepting their compliment. I'd recently heard a manners expert say it's impolite to speak about your problems while making small talk. I scribbled down:

· Be happier
· Maybe wear more pearls?

PEOPLE: Jess, I said I'm really happy for you.
ME: Thank you. I'm happy, too.

I felt like a fraud around friends, so I avoided hanging around the school, the park, and the local pool. (To be honest I stopped going to the pool when I started appearing on TV and was approached in the open concept showers by a superfan who wanted to know all about the biz while her kids curiously eyeballed my naked body.)

Yup. Home alone is the place for me!

The night before the show, when no one had told me otherwise, I figured I was actually going to be allowed to host. I slept at the InterContinental Hotel to ensure a smooth morning (one without kids rubbing toothpaste on my dress or asking rapid-fire questions like "What are teeth made of?" while I say, "I'm too busy to answer you," but really I never have answers and don't want my kids to feel insecure because their mom lacks general knowledge). A thousand other women had the same plan, and the hotel was booked to capacity. I guess we all called down for breakfast at the same time because there was a two-hour wait for eggs and toast. On an empty stomach I showered, straightened my hair, and slipped into a beautiful white silk sheath dress one of the sponsors had sent over (they don't do that when you work at a bank, I noted gratefully). I put on my nude five-inch heels and felt instantly important.

Look what's happening to Jessica Holmes… I mean, me!

Security (by this, I mean well-groomed guys in suits and earpieces) was abundant, and a good thing too because the audience was testy after hours of standing in line with no assigned seating. It was so chaotic that Oprah made an unplanned walk through the audience to make up for it, shaking hands and thanking people for their patience. It sort of backfired as people tumbled over each other to grab at her or snap frantic selfies or shout, "You are Jesus reincarnated," and security steered her backstage.

I watched it all on a monitor in the wings while I sipped coffee through a straw and ate packets of sugar because sugar is a form of food. Apparently, there was a whole green room somewhere, but I was trying to play it cool and look like I belonged and therefore couldn't bring myself to ask, "Hey, where are the snacks at?" Although Oprah's company was producing the televising of the event, a separate Canadian company was producing the live components, and I seemed to have fallen in the cracks between the two, other than one of the Chippendale-inspired security guards telling me, "Oprah and Céline Dion are friends, so don't use the Céline camel toe joke." I had a mouthful of sugar in that moment so I just nodded and gave a thumbs-up.

Finally, I was announced, and I danced onto the stage in front of 9,000 giddy Oprah fans, handing over the reins to my inner muse and committing to my act. I opened with a request that the audience take a deep yoga breath, hold it in, and "forgive the long lines" (which got a good laugh). I told jokes, did some impressions, and sang a song as Céline Dion, complete with the camel-toes chorus (sorry, sexy security guard, but it was too difficult to find an alternative rhyme for "paint your heart with my highs 'n' lows" on an empty stomach).

I felt relieved to finally be up there. My mind was so calm. Like when you jump into a lake and realize how quiet it is underwater. No what-ifs, no jealousy, no comfy sectionals to lie on while agonizing over wasted potential. None of it. I did a good job up there.

PAT: Wait, Jess, how can you still do comedy when you're an emotional robot?

ME: Right. Compartmentalization. Ok. Let's say that at ground zero (pre-depression), my week is comprised of the following standard schedule:

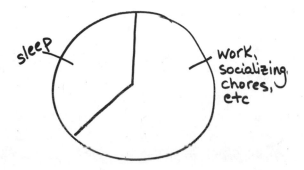

PAT: Oh. Wow. You know, there are some great apps out there to help you make pie charts.

ME: Neat! Forgot to mention that other artists probably have a generous pot-smoking slice of pie, too. Anyway, during my depression, my week was more like this:

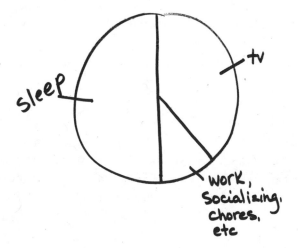

ME: I could always muster up the adrenalin and acting chops to be "on" for an hour on stage, but I would pay for it later by being an emotional zero for days. What a princess, right?
PAT: And your circles need work.
ME: Agree to disagree.

Overall it was an incredible show! World-renowned experts on self-actualization like Deepak Chopra and Iyanla Vanzant gave deep and charming insights into the soul. One of the guest speakers was Tony Robbins, a man whose thirty-day motivational cassettes (yes, cassettes!) had fuelled my early career success. After I introduced him, I came off stage and texted Scott to pick up celery if he got the chance. When the first show was finished, a new audience came in and we repeated the process. More jokes, more speakers, more sugar.

Four hours of feel-good anecdotes and hoopla later, the second show drew to a close. Security shooed everyone but me out of the backstage area.

And there she was.

The Oprah.

She walked off stage into the wings and stood twelve feet away from me in a beautiful red dress. Smiling at no one in particular, she slapped her hands on her hips with a satisfied exhale.

This is my moment!

I just stood there, looking at her like some hungry old-timey orphan staring into a pastry shop window. Paralyzed with insecurity. I wanted to at least say a polite "thank you,

Ms. Winfrey," but all I could muster up was "   ". A moment later her team whisked her away and she was gone.*

When I got home that night I looked up at my vision board, made years earlier with pictures of nature, musicals, Africa, veggies, and Oprah watching over it all like Glinda the Good Witch.

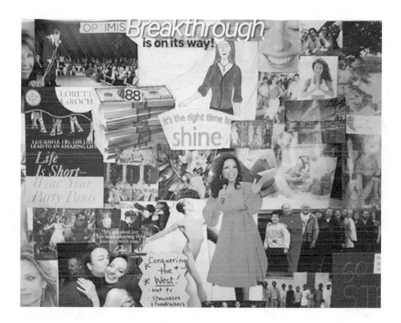

All my aspirations had materialized (except for the ridiculous ones like the stack of eighty-eight-dollar bills and the vegetables) and even now, with this new milestone under my belt, the most optimistic reaction I could summon was, again, neat.

---

* I later rationalized in a *Huffington Post* piece that I hadn't introduced myself because meeting her wouldn't trump all the inspiration she'd imparted over the years. I didn't know I was depressed when I wrote that.

I unfolded the list of takeaways I had jotted down that day, which were along the lines of:

If I just pull myself up by the bootstraps and focus on the positive and eat healthier and play with more kittens, then I can outrun this dark cloud.

I had written myself notes like this before, trying to keep up with Joneses of the smoothie-drinking, yoga-doing, list-completing crowd. Bucking up (and drinking coffee) could channel moments of fleeting motivation where I'd eat more celery and run around the block and focus desperately on the positive, but inevitably I'd land back on the sofa, feeling like a bigger failure than before. All the good advice in the world can't fix a funk when that funk is a depression.

But here's the great thing about us humans; whether we face great physical or emotional hardships, or like in my case, lose the will to dream, somewhere in the far corner of our minds, we still reckon something better *could* come along. There are times in life for lofty goals of success and creative fulfillment and self-actualization and making your own marshmallows or whatever other "favourite things" Oprah is championing. And then there are times when you need a simpler objective. Beneath my vision board, I taped up a new mantra—a placeholder, just till I felt less like a human turd. It's a line from Dory, when she's lost in *Finding Nemo*:

just
Keep
Swimming.

Miss Piggy

. . . . .

"**LIKE A ROTISSERIE** chicken" is the closest I can come to describing how I felt in Venezuela. I was there from '93 to '95 as a missionary spreading the gospel of the Church of Jesus Christ of Latter-day Saints, which is a fancy way of saying I went door to door being rejected for the Mormon church. We worked outside from 8 till 8 six days a week, on foot, wearing long rayon dresses, in blazing, unforgiving sun. When men would catcall us with a *tsssss-tsssss-tsssss* or a less subtle "Get over here, woman!" I remember thinking, "Wow, how do they have the energy in this heat? I mean, lust is evil, but their persistence is impressive!"

Despite being covered in greasy SPF 50 sunscreen, I was red-faced within an hour of the plane landing in Valencia, and the red didn't fade till I came back to Canada eighteen months later, only by then it was patchy and leathery. I was twenty-two years old and looked like I'd been wintering in Florida with the cotton-tops for decades.

PAT: Whoa, why didn't you just wear a hat, (dummy)?
ME: There was a strict no-hat policy because in Venezuela the only people who wear hats are farmers and no one wants to join a farm church.

PAT: What's a farm church?
ME: It's nothing. Look, just... read on.
PAT: M'kay.

Venezuelans gave me the nickname *la rojita*, which means "Little Red One." A lady we were trying to convert went so far as to describe me as looking like a tomato on a toothpick. (I showed her by gaining thirty pounds in my first eight months there and becoming more like a tomato on a zucchini. A *red* zucchini.) It was the kind of sunburn people describe as "angry." "Ooh, your skin looks angry," like it was so inflamed it could detach itself and enter a boxing ring at will. Actually, it would've been great if I could detach it. "Oh, that pock-y old thing? That's just the face I had in Venezuela. The one I'm wearing now is a newer model. It's from the Nicole Kidman line." Anyway...

Since part of being a missionary is looking approachable and not like you're leaving a burn unit, I had to buy concealer with the little spending money I had. At all times we were teamed up with another missionary, called a companion, and shared everything we had, including a bedroom. This made me extremely happy because I had always wanted a sister and had been reeling for a decade from my mom's refusal to birth me a playmate. She also turned down my request to adopt me a sister; "I called the adoption agency but they said we already had too many kids," which I realize now was a fib, but at least she did get me a girl cat named Midnight, who became my best friend and confidante, though we never shared clothes or braided each other's hair.

The companions switched every couple of months, so sometimes I had a "sister" who felt like a soul mate, and sometimes

I had a "sister" who annoyed me, as I've been told real sisters can do, so either way: winning! We got an allowance every month that was meant to cover food and transportation, and if there was anything leftover, you could use it on toiletries or souvenirs or clothing but I wouldn't recommend their clothing because anything made there had beads or embroidery on it and anything shipped over from North America had cartoon logos like Garfield or Popeye and, again, no one wanted to join an '80s cartoon church. The month that I started buying concealer, I ran out of money two days before the next allowance. At this time my companion was a stunningly beautiful woman who was not red but who also bought cosmetics and had run out of money. I called our Mission president and asked for a loan but was turned down "so you'll learn how to manage your finances." We didn't starve because we had powdered milk and dried kidney beans, which we ate for two days straight (separately, not as one recipe). My resentment built every time I farted unwittingly into the warm Venezuelan wind, thinking, "Guess what, Mission president? How approachable am I now?!" But, farts aside, I really did learn to manage money. Silver lining on a brown cloud.

The next month I bought a smaller bottle of makeup in a paler shade so that I could use less, because everyone knows if you mix ivory with red, you get light pink. Somehow concealer didn't work like oil paint and the ivory concealer just made me look like a vampire for the first part of the day, and by afternoon, when my cheeks sweated off the makeup, it looked like I was thawing back to life from a state of undead. People gushed over my beautiful companion with the almond eyes and Hollywood hair, then they'd see my face and say, "Ooooh that looks like it hurts."

It didn't upset me much because I wasn't hunting for romance in Venezuela (which wasn't allowed anyway). My facial shame came when I returned back to Canada, excited to find a Mormon husband within a year so that I wouldn't be considered totally over the hill at twenty-three and relegated to supervising dances and making sandwiches for the Sunday school kids, whose parents would quietly whisper to them, "Be nice to Sister Holmes. She has no one." But my being free-spirited and ruddy-faced was interpreted by my love interests as rowdy and weathered, so I remained single. On principle I didn't want any man who would reject me based on my risqué jokes or Florida face anyway. I remind my daughter daily (while I sheepishly spread globs of makeup on myself) that the only beauty that matters is on the inside.

My point is that I'm very cognizant of the sun's harmful rays, and I go to great lengths to shade my skin so I can continue to recover from a twenty-year-old sunburn. It's definitely made me a pain in the ass to makeup artists; "Can you get rid of the red? Actually, can you get rid of all the colour? You know what? Just make me look like I'm in a black-and-white film." Friends think I'm wearing hats and sunglasses because I want to be incognito, even though I've told them time and time again that I NEVER get recognized from my TV appearances unless I'm in some kind of compromising situation, like on a rushed morning when I haven't brushed my teeth or maybe I just sharted at Walmart. THAT is when someone stops me for a selfie.

PAT: Wow.
ME: Yup.

When I was in the thick of my depression, I'd look at my red face—pillow-creased and dehydrated—and feel like I was an atrocity. I already felt like I was botched on the inside, and it was reaffirmed when the outside matched. "If I'm too ugly for me, how can I NOT be too ugly for the rest of the world??" As the daughter of a feminist who didn't allow me to shave my legs or wear makeup until high school, when I became an adult I fell in love with the before-and-after "Ta-Da!" moment of my beauty ritual. But in my depressed state, any attempt at beauty seemed like a fraud; like I had put a fresh coat of varnish on a cracked doll. I'd slather on the makeup and do my hair (even going so far as getting long ratty yellow hair extensions glued to the base of my real hair to cover up the extra pounds I couldn't shed).

No one will notice my face or body if I have straw-like doll hair sticking out from beneath my real hair.

It just made me look as desperate as I felt. I started calling myself Miss Piggy when I looked in the mirror.

Yup, chubby cheeks, yellow locks, Tammy Faye Bakker lashes, and too much blush... I look like Miss Piggy... if Miss Piggy was an old escort.

"How can anyone love me?" I'd ask the cat, who ignored my question and gnawed aggressively at her foot. The deeper I got into my depression, the uglier I felt and the harder I tried to fix my feelings with external Band-Aids, like online shopping. When I had a burst of energy, instead of using it in a productive way like organizing my desk, starting up a writing project, or socializing, I used it to feverishly shop online. At least once a week, I'd browse for hours and hours, thinking "if I could just find the right outfit, it would take away all my insecurities." I'd get packages of eccentric, colourful rock-star clothes I didn't need and *definitely* couldn't pull off unless I was working on a Canadian remake of *Sex and the City*. (What would that be called anyway? *Sex and the Sorry? Snow and the City?* Meh—I'll keep working on it.) Returning the outfits meant walking to the post office, which I couldn't do 'cause of, well, no good reason. Despite our line of credit growing irresponsibly large, I gave the items to friends, or stuck them in a wobbly pile Scott dropped off monthly to charity. If you're ever at Value Village and you see a gold bodysuit or pleather dress with the tags still attached, you're welcome!

Fast-fix beauty rituals were another pick-me-up I tried, but I'm extremely cheap, and instead of going to an actual dermatologist for help with my complexion, I got an online discount deal for laser therapy at a "spa" in the wrong part of town, where some lady wearing flip-flops squirted baby oil on me, then ironed my face with a large metal wand. It caused my rosacea to flare up like a baboon's bottom. The only answer was another online discount deal. This time—

PAT: No! The answer was not another online discount deal! The answer was to love yourself for who you are.

ME: Well, sure, tell me that now!

This time it was for a tanning salon in the wrong part of town. I arrived wearing a thick scarf around my blotchy face (despite it being summer), and pulled it down to tell the Goth teenager behind the desk I was here for my appointment.

HER: Your lady didn't show up today. I'll do it.

ME: Oh. (*pause*) Ok. I'm pale everywhere but my face, so can I get a spray tan for light or fair complexions?

HER: No. We just have one colour for everyone.

ME: Oh. So, heh-heh, basically everyone comes out looking like Jennifer Aniston?

HER: (*angry Goth stare*)

I stepped into a slippery booth, naked except for a shower cap, and Goth-girl sprayed me half-heartedly while she picked at her chipped nail polish. The machine was temperamental and made a sputtering sound every so often as it ran out of spray. I looked down and noticed that it was not, in fact, making me look like a body double for J.Lo but a brown-and-white Dalmation.

ME: I think you missed a spot.

HER: Where.

ME: Everywhere.

HER: Well, rub it around. I got a pedicure coming in two minutes.

I rubbed, and looked in the mirror.

What have I done?!

Despite Goth-girl missing half of my body, she sure didn't miss my face! I looked like Tan Mom from the neck up. I jumped in the changeroom shower and frantically scrubbed every inch of my body, but it just went from dark brown blotchy to medium brown blotchy. I tenderly dabbed at my raw face, but barely any colour came off on the washcloth, leaving me with the original red *plus* a new brown topcoat. I paid and thanked and tipped Goth-girl (because I have zero assertiveness skills) and held back my tears till I got to the car.

It can't be as bad as I think. It can't be as bad
as I think. It can't be as bad as I think.

I took a selfie of my winningest smile, then sent the pic to my best friend Genna hoping she'd tell me, "It's fine," just like she had on all those other occasions when I got bad discount highlights, bad discount brow shaping, and bad discount hair extensions. This time, she replied, "Oh, honey, you look like a brown turtle."

And that, Pat, is when I stopped buying online discount deals.

PAT: Good!

ME: Yup.

PAT: You should just be yourself.

ME: Yup.

PAT: ... can I see the selfie?

ME: Nope.

Years later, after recovering from depression, I realized the only beauty ritual guaranteed to make me feel marvellous is exercise. Sometimes, after a long run or a soccer game, I'll catch myself in the mirror and think, "Huh. I'd tap that." Beyond that, the only beauty advice I have is:

wear sunscreen.

I am still very protective of my skin, especially on holidays. You know how big celebrities summer in the Hamptons? Little celebrities summer in a trailer park. We have a thirty-eight-foot Golden Falcon park model plunked on a quiet lake in the middle of Nowhere, Ontario. When I hit the beach, I pack protective swimwear and hats big enough to obstruct people's view. One day I tripped coming out of the water, and my friend commented to his wife, "Oh my god, look at that old nurse caught in the waves," before realizing it was just me. Yes, maybe swimming in a white SPF 50 long-sleeved shirt and matching full-length pants doesn't make me the next Sofia Vergara, but you bet your buns, if the Irish-Canadian Cultural Society put out a discount swimsuit calendar, I'd be invited to pose as the pale centrefold in the summer-weight turtleneck.

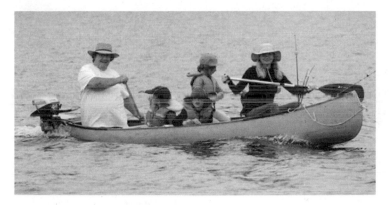

Riding in a "Canadian yacht" (a canoe with a motor attached to it) with my dad and some young 'uns. Photo courtesy of Scott, who I think might have taken it in a spirit of mockery.

My point is, it feels so good to be in a place where my insecurities don't torment me, where looking like an old nurse instead of a Bond girl on the beach doesn't send me into an online shopping panic, but rather lets me revel in my happy place, being the butt of the joke. So I'm sorry, Value Village, I'm keeping the sun hats and cover-all swimsuits for myself.

Marriage Is So Fun for the First Couple of Years!

* * * * *

I HAVEN'T SPOKEN much of my husband, Scott, yet. Not because I'm hiding anything. He's not hiding anything either (I know because I've looked in his journal). When I asked if I could mention him in the book, he said, "Well, what exactly..." but that's all I heard because I could tell by the look on his face he would've said yes and I didn't really want to stand there like a dummy while he finished his sentence so I ran back here to start writing about love.

ME: *Doodly-doodly-doodly*—
PAT: Another flashback?
ME: You betcha!

EXT. ARTS HIGH SCHOOL. DAY.
We pan across a field where teens are sitting in groups: punks, jocks, nerds. Jessica sits near a group of artsies playing hacky sack. Several of them have cold sores. She is wearing a Cosby sweater and a miniskirt. She stares longingly at a group of boys vandalizing a car.

In the fall of 1987 I woke up one day obsessed with boys. But much like in a rom com, I had to get some misconceptions about romance out of the way before I was ready to fall for the right guy. I had seen *Grease* way too young and learned that the leading man doesn't want some tramp—he wants the nice girl whose simple goal in life is to be sweet so that he can *turn* her into a tramp, and that's what makes their car fly. Girl good + boy bad = love. I guess that movie kind of imprinted on me, and gave me a warped sense of what's romantic; like if the first thing a newly hatched duckling were to see was a human, it would mimic the human behaviour. Sweet life for a duck, though: TV dinners, playing on the iPad, sleeping indoors on Egyptian cotton shee—

PAT: Jess?
ME: Right!

I dated in high school, but only the bad boys. A punk, then a skinhead, then, I don't know, I couldn't find anyone more bad than a skinhead.

PAT: You know "more bad" isn't correct?
ME: I do now—thanks!

When I followed in my father's footsteps and became Mormon at eighteen, I was disappointed to learn that there really wasn't a bad boy in the church. Sure, there was one who wore a three-button suit instead of a two-button suit and that made the herd a little jittery, but not a lot of Mormon James Deans.

It's not a choice every teenager would make, to shut the party down just when it's getting good, but going to an arts high school allows you to get the drinking/sexual exploring phase out of the way early. And I'd been impressed with the peacefulness I felt when I visited my dad's church over the years. (My agnostic mom rolled her eyes when I told her about it. Not sure how their marriage is so good when he thinks after death she won't make it to heaven and she thinks after death he'll just decompose.) By the time I graduated I'd started thinking, "I need to clean this party up!" A year later, near the end of a three-month backpacking trip through Europe with my friend Tara, I had an epiphany. We were leaving yet another bar having tried yet another beer and flirted with yet another [insert nationality here], and I felt like I had reached the peak of adolescence. It's like there was a list of stupid things you're supposed to accomplish to ace "Bad Teenager 101" and I had checked off the minimum number of required boxes to move forward.

- ☐ Sneaking liquor from babysitting clients (sorry about watering down your vodka, Mr. and Ms. Weathers!)
- ☐ Stealing from my parents and defending my behaviour with "It's your fault for not locking up your stuff!"
- ☐ Smoking tea leaves (friends told me it was marijuana, then busted me when I wheezed, "I definitely feel something")
- ☐ Forging my parents' signatures so I could play hooky (yup, I got caught)

Dear Sir or Madam,
Please excuse Jessica from
School today due to stuff.
Sincerely, ~~mom and dad~~
her parents.

Perhaps it was divine inspiration or homesickness or a chance to wash away regrets, but coming out of a bar in Amsterdam I turned to Tara and said, "I think I'm gonna be a Mormon." Tara, who was mellow from pot but also mellow in general, squinted at me, then shrugged. "Well, they have good dances."

They do *have good dances. Decision made!*

Within a few days of returning home I informed my joyous father and disappointed mother of the great news.

ME: Guess what, guys? I'm joining the Mormon church!
DAD: That's just great. Welcome aboard!
MOM: Nooooooooo!

Mother is a feminist, you see. A full-blown, short-haired, makeup-free advocate for positive change for womYn. This new church I loved, with a reputation for having (sweeping generalization alert) men at the helm while women were encouraged to be righteous, kind, and handy with preservatives, doesn't jive with all crowds.

ME: They're such good people, Mom! And you'll just die when you try these canned pears!
MOM: Jess, how can you reconcile their beliefs with your own values?
ME: Don't sweat it, Mom. God's got my back. And He could have yours, too! In fact, I've been meaning to share this book with you. It's called the Book of M—
MOM: No! No! No! No!

Though I severed ties with my exes, cleaned up my language ("f#$k" became "darn" and "sh&thead" became "silly-billy"), and replaced miniskirts with flowing rayon dresses, I couldn't get a date among the new fold. At our church, there was a tall, handsome family where every kid was better-looking than the last. The Harpers (name changed 'cause maybe I still have a chance with one of them in the afterlife and a clever gal hedges her bets) had toothy Kennedy smiles and solid square jaws. Even the women! They were tall and self-assured. Normally I'd resent this level of goody-two-shoe'dness but they were disarmingly kind and inclusive and told stories of their fun adventures that made you want to marry into the clan or at least develop a G-rated sitcom around them.

> *"Thursdays at 8, tune in to The Harpers!*
> *The Harpers: their hearts are*
> *as grand as their teeth!"*

I tried to woo every Harper within three years of my age: I dressed prettier and spoke more politely and averted my eyes coquettishly when one of them shared a hymnal with me (unfortunately that's not a metaphor for anything), but, still, no dice.

So I brushed myself off and set my sights on the Wilsons (name also changed to keep afterlife prospects open), an upstanding set of rosy-cheeked twins. When that yielded nothing I moved on to the Bundys, the Cunninghams, and the Seavers. Dead ends.

It might have been my grown-out perm, which I'd recently dyed burgundy;

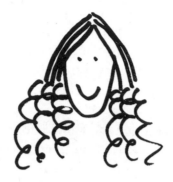

my odd choice of small talk ("cat kibble is just as salty as it looks"); or the fact that my mother wasn't a member, making me some kind of half-heathen. I realized that I was a 5 in Mormonia despite being a 7 anywhere else—maybe even a 7.5 in England, where my pointy nose would fit in better? Whatever the cause, no fish were biting.

PAT: I don't get it. What was the rush?

ME: Uh, waiting to be married to have sex was the rush. And considering my local church only had about twenty eligible bachelors, I felt that desperately chasing boys was my only play.

PAT: That's a terrible play!

ME: With terrible results!

Hitting on a guy when you're also trying to pass yourself off as subservient is tough, complicated work. I was clearly failing at it because after two years of my sneakily aggressive advances, no one had requited my love except for one friend who was hoping to skip over that whole dating thing:

HIM: I've prayed, and you're to be my wife.

ME: Uh... (*squinting for twelve seconds*) I just prayed and got a different answer.

At a dance that summer, while I stood alone with arms crossed, staring resentfully at the girls whose hair wasn't a grown-out burgundy perm, whose blouses weren't taken in at the back so their breasts would be more prominent, who weren't chewing gum and telling stories ending in "then the guy farts!", I realized... *I* was the bad boy.

This is no place for a screwball like me.

The first few dates I got after leaving the church were with—

PAT: Hey, you sort of skipped over a whole chunk. Are you going to elaborate on leaving a religion behind?
ME: Nah. We're skipping dinner to get straight to dessert. Roll with it!
PAT: Guess I have no choice.
ME: That's the spirit!

—were with milquetoast* "okely dokely" guys you might meet at a craft fair who invite you to move in with them at their grandma's on the second date. I was on fire since I had found comedy and was looking for more of an adventure than raising squirrels in Guelph, Ontario. (No disrespect to those who raise squirrels in Guelph, Ontario. I'm sure it's a wholesome, rewarding life!) When I ran into Scott at a comedy club, he might as well have been standing in a beam of light shining

---

* A funner way of saying unassertive. I promise that's the only five-dollar word in the book!

down from heaven. He was charismatic, but with a very positive twist, like a young George Bailey from *It's a Wonderful Life*. I had first met Scott at Ryerson University back in my churchy days when I was a student and he was working at the school's audio-visual lab. I had an immediate crush on him, but I couldn't find the nerve to strike up a conversation, which is ok because at the time I was training to become a missionary and my pickup line might have been "Have you heard about the time Christ came to America?" But now, years later, I was footloose and religion-free! We talked for an hour after the show; that giddy, crushy talk about what your favourite food is and what music you like and anything else elementary enough to be understood while shouted over The Proclaimers' "500 Miles."

The next day Genna (whose boyfriend was one of Scott's roommates) called to say he had asked her for my number.

GENNA: Don't hurt him, Jessie.
ME: Huh? Why would I do that?
GENNA: He's really, really nice. Like, a really kind person.
ME: I like nice guys.
GENNA: (*silence*)
ME: What? I do. That guy Steve wasn't my fault! He was always quoting Homer Simpson and promising, "Someday I'll take you to the top of the CN tower," like I was his kid. Totally not my fault.
GENNA: I guess.
ME: (*gushing*) Oh my gosh, Genna, he's so tall!
GENNA: Yeah. And he's really quirky. Like, he bought this really cool purple sofa. It's velvet and has this beige piping—
ME: He owns his own sofa? Not a futon? Oh my gosh, he's rich!

GENNA: (*sighing*) Oh Jess. Wow. No. He lives with three roommates next to Hooker Harvey's. I was just trying to point out how cool he is and—

ME: Have you seen his hair? It's, like, really nice.

GENNA: Oh lord. You're gonna hurt him.

ME: I won't! This isn't like Carlos with the small hands, I swear. I have a good feeling.

And I didn't hurt him. Not for a long time.

PAT: So, you were mentally healthy back then?

ME: I prefer the term "pre-loopy." But, yes, I finished the mission in Venezuela a few years earlier, and even though I had left the church, I still felt the excited ambition of a woman with everything ahead of her. Not a jaded bone in my body. I was working days at an obscure branch of the government, and reading self-actualization books on the subway every night on my way to comedy clubs.

PAT: Wow, busy much?

ME: Not really. The office I worked at was a snooze-fest. One day my boss pulled me aside and said: "You're too ambitious to work here. Seriously, look around." I looked around at the folks playing solitaire, the guy who only worked 10 to 2, the woman who spent the day fighting on the phone with her boyfriend, the guy who snacked on baby carrots non-stop. But it was an easy place to work where I could jot down funny ideas and relax.

PAT: Your boss didn't mind?

ME: Nah, chronic napper.

PAT: Oh.

I was at work when I first got the call from Scott. I had to block one ear so I could concentrate over the baby-carrot-devouring one cubicle over. It happened to be my birthday, and Scott serenaded me while accompanying himself on the guitar.

A normal guy is flirting with me!

On our first date, he took me to a cavernous restaurant on Yonge Street that had red velvet wallpaper and big portions of so-so food. The kind of place a twenty-four-year-old who had only eaten at chip wagons and Duff's Smorgasbord in Ottawa would call "really high end." I thought it was charming that Scott's plaid shirt was tucked snug into his jeans and that he carried a man purse with an old-fashioned umbrella swinging from it. "Forecast says 30 percent chance of rain," he announced. I had gotten my hair cut and highlighted in a blond newscaster bob. I caught our reflection and thought that we made a clean-cut pair, the kind of couple you see applying for a first mortgage in a bank commercial.

See? I can be the nice girl.

Here we are!

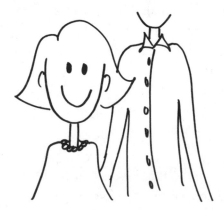

PAT: Where's his head?

ME: Oops. He's really tall and it was hard to fit him in. Here, there he is.

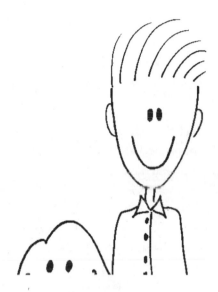

PAT: Uh...

ME: I know—cute couple, right?!

He spoke about his experiences as an actor and I was completely in awe, having just started in the business.

ME: I'm taking classes at Second City.* And I'm the door girl at the Laugh Resort. But my agent told me, "Just do your show and leave. You don't want to get in that dark place."

SCOTT: You don't strike me as dark.

ME: Oh I'm not. I'm, like, super happy all the time. But I

---

* Cool people leave out the "The."

guess that's her point, to stay happy. She had a friend in the business who nearly overdosed. Do you do drugs?

SCOTT: God, no. Never even smoked pot.

ME: Yay. (*clapping hands*)

A mouse ran across the railing next to our table, and we both laughed at how cute it was. He insisted on paying the bill, which I appreciated because he was a game show host after all.

PAT: Wait, a game show host?

ME: Yes! Can you believe it? If I played my cards right, I could be the wife of a game show host! I probably sound like a gold digger, but you have to understand I had waited years for a real date... *And* I was living in a shared rental behind the bus terminal.

PAT: (*crossing arms*) There it is.

ME: Do you know how trippy your dreams get when you hear "last call for Wawa" mid-sleep? Plus, I didn't want to be the third wheel again when I visited my family, being driven in the backseat like an eight-year-old while relatives cock their heads sadly to the side and ask, "Have you met anyone?"

PAT: Hm. I see—so for all the wrong reasons, you wanted this to work.

ME: And one right reason. L—

PAT: Oh, don't say it.

ME: Love.

PAT: Wow.

ME: Yeah.

We walked fifteen blocks up Yonge Street while he told me about each of his past relationships.

SCOTT: ...and I had this habit of being an emotional handyman, and my therapist thought I should st—

ME: Uh, I'm totally appreciating your "I'm an open book" approach, but maybe you could save these over-shares for a time that *isn't* our first date?

SCOTT: Oh. Of course! I'm just so happy to be out with you I'm rambling!

ME: And what's an emotional handyman?

SCOTT: Well, that's a dynamic where—

ME: Actually, never mind. Wanna catch a movie?

We ducked into a theatre and watched *Return to Paradise*—a painful, excruciating movie about a man imprisoned in Malaysia. It was a tear-jerker, but when I reached into my purse for a tissue, I pulled out a handful of old tattered ones, along with some remarkably large lint balls and old candy wrappers. Scott offered me one of his clean, neatly folded tissues.

Classy!

When the credits rolled, he laughingly declared it "worst first-date movie, ever!" We walked to a nearby friend's apartment where I was house-sitting and I pondered inviting him in for [grown-up stuff]. In front of the building there was a decorative boulder. I stood up on it, thinking it would make it easier for Scott, who I thought might be eight feet tall, to kiss me. Instead he winked at me and walked away whistling. I stood on the boulder like a meerkat and watched him go. Despite the restaurant being terrible, the movie being gut-wrenching, and him only actually being six-foot-five, I was intrigued.

Well, that was neat!

On our next date, all I got was a peck on the cheek. And on our third date, when I walked him home in the rain, I got one heck of a kiss, but he didn't invite me in. "Good things are worth waiting for," he said as he slowly closed the door on me. I tapped on his window with my umbrella till his landlord came out and I ran off like a sneaky pervert.

Playing hard-to-snuggle paid off for him, and I proposed to Scott two years later when it struck me that he was so much more than a boyfriend. (I had started referring to him as my life partner the year before but his father thought that sounded too big-city-pretentious so instead I just called him "my lover" around family). "If we get married, I'll have him tied up," I thought, like a husband was something you corral. Sometimes when I'm feeling insecure and crushing anxiety is making me think I'm not planted firmly enough, I look at all I've amassed: two kids, awesome friends, an RV, a few fancy shoes, and a Scott. "Phew, I've paired up and put down roots. I'm not just going to float away into space!"

If we had met online, we likely wouldn't have been a match.

My profile:
- Busy mind with no off switch
- Feels she's right 100 percent of the time, but gripes about it privately, as she fears confrontation
- Considers salad a main course
- Thrill-seeker
- Plans on cleaning up after herself someday, just not now

Scotty's:
- Doesn't sweat small stuff
- Feels that everyone is always right because each soul has its own truth, and therefore doesn't believe in confrontation

- Thinks people are kidding when they order salad as a main course
- Peacekeeper
- Hobbies include dishwashing and saving people

An expert in the field of mental health may have looked at this match and said, "I'm not supposed to speak in these terms, but basically she's nuts and he's an enabler and she's gonna destroy him."

This nut/enabler dynamic is perhaps why, when my depression was at its worst, we hadn't really discussed what was wrong with me. I alternated between being furious and apologizing; anger, guilt, anger, guilt—over and over. There was no in-between place to get close. We had two kids by then, and I rationalized my behaviour as "just part of the early years." Most mornings I would declare hopefully, "Today is the day we start fresh," and then I'd trip over Scott's long shoes and snap, "There's too much crap in this house! I can't be the cleaner, the parent, the cook, and the comedian! I can't handle this!"

"I can't handle this" had become my mantra, even though we actually had a delightful nanny who helped with cooking and cleaning, so my rantings were inaccurate on top of hysterical. And perhaps that's why I avoided opening up to my friends. They tried to be supportive but they were also confused because I *shouldn't* be unwell. They had tangible problems: a breakup, a layoff, a kid who bites. My problems were invisible and/or unrelatable. Something as innocuous as an empty tissue box could trigger a full Donald Duck–grade meltdown: "Kleenex is a couple bucks a box. Why the f#$k do we not have boxes and boxes and boxes of tissue in every room?!" All that was missing was cartoon steam shooting out of my ears. Fun times. Ugh. No wonder Scott and I had zero intimacy.

In my defence, I got the impression no parents of kids under five were doing it. I was part of a moms' group that met once a week to discuss children and recipes and how we read somewhere that plastic will make mutants of future generations. One week we decided to do a marital satisfaction survey where we and our significant others filled in a questionnaire without showing each other, evaluating our relationship in several categories like friendship, finance, housekeeping, and making whoopee. One fabulously energetic mom compiled all the results based on gender and came up with this summary:

Women's suggestions:	Men's suggestions:
• Fill me up a bubble bath	• Touch my junk more
• Look deep into my eyes	
• Surprise me with candles, flowers, or chocolate (only the organic, dark, fair-trade kind)	
• Show more of an interest in my pottery hobby. Don't just call every mug I make "neat." Learn some new adjectives!	

I was secretly relieved that husbands were unanimously not getting any.

PAT: Well, they didn't say they weren't getting any, just that they wanted more.

ME: Pat, c'mon. They weren't getting any so they were just like my husband.

PAT: But that doesn't—
ME: I can't hear you. *LA-LA-LA-LA*—
PAT: Forget it. Carry on.

I didn't touch junk, like, ever. This was a shame because when Scott and I are intimate, it's pretty great. I knew if we fast-forwarded from me angrily watching TV to me in bed with him, we'd, how shall I put this... we'd all walk away winners.

PAT: Way to stay classy!
ME: Thanks. I was gonna write, "We'd get our freak on," but
I took it out 'cause I'd never want my parents to read that!
PAT: Uh, you know you just—

But I couldn't get from A to B; couldn't stand the thought of letting the wall down. It felt too vulnerable, like touching him was some kind of admission that he wasn't my enemy in other areas. So I just closed up shop. This left Scott in the uncomfortable position of feeling like a jerk if he pressured me (and his version of pressure is "I don't mind waiting—but can you please tell me roughly how long I'll be waiting? Is it like a month or are we talking years? 'Cause I'm not gonna wait *years*. (*pause*) I take that back. I didn't mean to go all berserk there. I'd *prefer* to not wait years, please"), and livin' la vida eunuch if he didn't. When the kids were in the room, we had an unspoken rule that we'd be especially nice to each other, even hugging, with both of us eyeing the kids to see if they had seen Mommy and Daddy's display of love, and did they look convinced?

That February my GP was away so I went to a walk-in clinic to renew a thyroid prescription. The doctor, an older woman who spoke slowly with a dignified eastern European accent, seemed to have no interest in efficiency and spoke at length about her daughter who lived in Florida while I lounged on the crunchy paper of the examination table. I figured if she could ignore the fact that there were four patients waiting to see her after me, I could, too. I wedged open the door to the place where my feelings used to be and opened up.

ME: I'm not sure if there's something wrong with me or not, but I don't feel like having sex with my husband.

DOCTOR: The best thing about being a woman is that you can pretend to like it, and no one will know.

ME: That's the BEST thing about being a woman?

DOCTOR: If a man can't have a woman naturally, he might just take her.

ME: Whoa, uh, I can't really see my husband doing that. He's kind of a pacifist. And he bruises easily.

DOCTOR: It's best to just lie there and it's done.

ME: For sure. For sure. Thanks. So, if I could just get this prescription filled, I'll be on my way.

I pulled on my coat, madly looking around in my peripheral vision to see any certification on the wall.

The spouses of people in my predicament often withdraw and have affairs, get a divorce, or suffer quietly through it out of love or loyalty or lack of a good exit strategy. That night Scott came into my room (he had moved to the spare bedroom a few years earlier when his snoring started to register on the Richter scale) and hovered uncomfortably. I decided to offer him a life raft. I slowly exhaled and closed my well-worn copy of *Outlander*, but as usual couldn't find one of the fifty bookmarks my children made me among the disarray on the nightstand, and ended up just reaching for one of the scraps on the pile, which in this case turned out to be a Band-Aid still in its package. I placed it in the book and turned to him. "I'm giving you a hall pass," I said.

If you don't happen to have a seedy vocabulary, you'll be surprised to know a hall pass refers to a person giving their partner permission to get nookie elsewhere.

SCOTT: Is this a trap?

ME: Seriously. I won't get mad. I need fewer things on my to-do list and this would really take the pressure off. Please just say yes.

SCOTT: I'm not interested in—

ME: Done! You are as free as a bird. Wow, I feel better already. This is good.

SCOTT: But, but, Jess . . .

ME: Sorry, babe, but I had planned to power-watch a bunch of shows on the iPad. So if I could be alone, that would be great. So glad we resolved this!

The further my pendulum swung to an unacceptable place, the further his acceptance swung with it. Maybe my devolution from civilized woman to angry couch-rodent was so gradual that he didn't feel the shock he should have. But there we were.

THAT SPRING, DESPITE my belief that leaving the house was for emergencies only, Scott convinced me to audition for a small recurring role on a tween comedy series. At the audition I was so foggy-headed that I could barely get through a sentence without staring down at the script, lost again and again. You know when your eyes sort of get stuck on one object, and even when you try to pull your gaze away, it stays there for a moment, almost like you're hypnotized? Lately I had noticed that sensation around the clock. And despite adrenalin and

coffee, I was now experiencing this fogginess even while performing. I started using familiar material from years earlier
("Here's my impression of the Spice Girls, wearing Crocs,
shopping for Beanie Babies") so I could be on autopilot on
stage, and not bother with improvisation because I couldn't
find the words to express what I meant. I asked Scott to start
accompanying me to local jobs so he could help me go over
material pre-show and make me feel better post-show if I had
messed up, like at a recent charity auction where I acted as
the auctioneer:

ME: Do I hear 450? Yes, 450 over here. Now, who will up the
   bid to 400?
AUDIENCE: (*discontented grumble*)
ME: Oh, sorry, what was the last bid?
AUDIENCE: 450!
ME: Right! Of course. Who will bring us up to 325?
AUDIENCE: 500!
ME: Really? Just a sec, I'm gonna start writing the numbers
   down.

Scott found all the right words to make me feel like a bit
less of a loser: "It could happen to anyone"; "I'm sure no one
noticed"; "Math isn't everyone's strong suit." I went in for a
rare no-kid-spectator hug, and Scott squeezed me tight. "It's
ok, Jess. None of this matters." I tried so hard to believe him.

He wasn't able to accompany me on a job to the ski town
of Whistler for a paper company event, but I figured it was no
big deal because I was only doing thirty minutes of comedy.
No auctioning, no math. On the drive up from the airport, the
client said, "Whatever you do, don't mention their competi-
tor: Kleenex. Say tissue if you have to."

Don't say Kleenex. Don't say Kleenex. Don't say Kleenex.

I referred to Kleenex in the first five minutes on stage. I heard a gasp in the audience and knew I'd screwed up. On my ride back to the airport with the client, I already couldn't remember whether it was Kleenex or some other brand I wasn't supposed to say, so I just kept quiet. I was humiliated by my mental incompetence over and over; I showed up to a sound check for a Tim Hortons event drinking from a Starbucks cup. The event planner grabbed the cup out of my hand and tossed it in the garbage, muttering "What are you thinking?!" under his breath. At their agency's party a few summers later, after I'd recovered from depression, I was in conversation with a new employee who was musing about the challenges of event planning. I asked, "Like what?" 'cause I love me some stories, and he proceeded to share anecdotes of clients showing up drunk, or the power going out mid-show, followed by "and before I came onboard here, apparently some comedian shows up to a Timmy's gig with a Starbucks. I would have fired them on the spot." His boss quickly changed the conversation and I laughed as though I didn't know who he'd been talking about.

PAT: Did you get that part?
ME: What part? Oh, right! The tween series audition!

So I was fumbling through the lines, and the look on the director's face said, "Are you having a stroke?" but what came out of her mouth was "Did you not get these lines beforehand?" I struggled to find an excuse that wasn't "I don't know who I am or what's wrong with me" and blurted out, "My kids were up all night with the flu. I'm operating on zero sleep."

They hired me (exclusively based on my previous experience, I assume) and it felt so good to be part of a team again. To set the alarm, shower, and be responsible for showing up somewhere every day.

I know what's expected of me and how to do it.

Every morning while my hair and makeup were done, I let go of my own worries and eavesdropped on the young cast's conversations about how gluten is basically Satan and which celebrities wore toupées (apparently, it's all of them). I struggled with memorization and was responsible for many a fifth take, but at least my new routine made me feel less like a human dust bunny. A week into the month-long shoot, Scott was driving me to set and a friend of his called to ask whether we'd like to invest in a movie he was making. It was an indie comedy that just needed bridge financing (a loan to carry the production until government funding comes through) to the tune of $150,000, which we were guaranteed to get back a year later after earning interest on the loan.

PAT: Oh Jess, no.

ME: Well, Scott said he was a great guy, really solid...

PAT: I feel sick.

ME: ... and that bridge financing was a sure thing. And we'd earn $2,000 a month in interest. We had actually run out of money, and had racked up debt between the nanny's salary and my online shopping, so it made twice as much sense.

PAT: No, that makes it lunacy.

ME: But the bank had an "unlimited refill" attitude toward lines of credit!

PAT: This is bad.

ME: I really needed a pick-me-up.

PAT: So get a puppy!

ME: Well, yes. In hindsight a puppy would have been cheaper.

I had a sick feeling in my stomach, a real NO of a feeling. And then the guy on the phone said, "And of course with that investment you'll be credited as an executive producer." My ego flooded me with the memories of how good it felt to be on top, to feel important, to get swag bags filled with branded pens and mugs, even though you put them in the "take me, I'm free" box at next summer's garage sale. My energy had picked up with this tween series, I was finally starting to feel like more than a puddle of misery, and I was terrified of losing this momentum.

I said yes because I was desperate and depressed.

Scott said yes because he likes helping his friends out— you know, helping someone move, being a shoulder to cry on, impersonating a bank...

The next day we took out the money on a line of credit, and it really was as easy as getting a slushy refilled at the corner store. But that night was the first of many when I would lie awake with an uneasy feeling about our debt, and try to brush it away by pulling a pillow over my face and picturing a peaceful scene: being on a train, passing under a starry night, the rumbling of the engine and creaking of the wheels against the rails, in a giant berth, with Scott spooning me, me spooning Alexa, Alexa spooning Jordan, and Jordan spooning our cat. It worked well enough, and an hour or two later I'd fall back to sleep. Train visualization stopped working when the loan became overdue by a year, then two. By then I'd be awake from roughly 2 to 5:30 each night (well, morning), playing emotional whack-a-mole, trying to beat back the panic that kept popping up in reasonable and useless concerns alike:

What if the bank wasn't joking when they told us to pay off our debt?

Where would we go if we lost the house? The trailer park only accepts residents May through October!!

Why is John Stamos peddling yogourt?

One morning I was still tossing and turning at 5:45, desperate to fall back asleep because I had a show that night. I wanted to be held and squeezed, like in one of Temple Grandin's cow-calming machines. I tiptoed to Scott's room, moved Suzan (his body pillow) out of the way, and backed up against him so I was the little spoon.

ME: Tell me everything is ok.
SCOTT: Everything *is* ok. Everything is great.
ME: Even if we have to go live under an underpass?
SCOTT: You're back on the homeless thing again, huh? (*sigh*) We'd still be okay.
ME: I'm sorry I'm awful.
SCOTT: No, honey, you're amazing. I love you so much.
ME: Ok.

I got up and moved the garbage can into the hall in front of Scott's door, a signal the kids knew meant "sleeping in, do not disturb." I crawled back in with Scott and slept.

"Mommy!" the kids yelled when I walked down the stairs around 8, and I was relieved to shift the focus off myself. We joked and kissed and laughed until Scott left with them for the schoolyard. I walked down to the basement and tried to fall back to sleep on the blue sofa. A few minutes later Scott returned, and, thinking we were now best buddies because of his heroic cuddling during the night, sat down beside me. He reached out to touch my leg, and I recoiled.

A little part of me wishes I could have warned him back on that first date that those were mentally healthy years for me, and that eventually it would start going downhill. But I'm sure if he tallied up all my tantrums and resentment, he'd still say it was worth it. Because he's just that nice.

Unable to help myself, I sighed angrily. "What is it? I'm busy." He stared at his hands and said, "I think we need marriage counselling."

Ugh.

Sorry, Pat—what a downer. Things get brighter in the next chapter, but here's a picture of a bunny in the meantime.

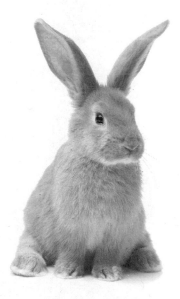

It Takes a Village
to Save a Marriage

. . . . .

A FRIEND OF mine once described her volatile marriage to me like this: "Marriage is a marathon, not a sprint. We might take a few losses in the short term, but in the long run I'm gonna cross the finish line with the love of my life!" I thought it was amazing advice, and didn't discredit it just because she divorced that guy a year later. Scott and I are good marathoners, I think. We're both early to bed, early to rise; we both love shopping for books we probably won't read; we're content to spend the summer at a trailer park; and we both like soup. Actually, we're gonna make terrific senior citizens! Where we blow chunks is the day-to-day. We don't win many sprints.

Scott's a fixer (I was going to couch it by calling him a nurser, but I think that might mean something else entirely and I'm not sure he'd begrudge it any less). On our first Valentine's Day together, he bought me the book *Don't Sweat the Small Stuff*. I smiled at the gift.

That's so Scott!

I unwrapped the second gift, which was obviously going to be the REAL gift, but instead it was the *Don't Sweat the Small Stuff Workbook*. I was confused because neither of these gifts contained sugar.

ME: Totally grateful! Just curious why I'm getting these for Valentine's Day?

SCOTT: I wanted to give you something useful.

ME: Oh, cool, well, maybe they'd make better gifts on a different holiday. Like if I got these on St. Patrick's Day, I'd probably be like: "These supersede my expectations!"

I didn't want to seem ungrateful, and pondered, "What would Jesus do?" He would accept them. But I doubted he'd actually fill in the workbook, what with his busy schedule and bell-sleeved robe getting in the way. I contemplated "don't look a gift horse in the mouth" versus "always be honest" and then kind of got sidetracked wondering why people would tell you to avoid looking at horse teeth when the better advice is probably "don't sniff a horse in the mouth, gifted or otherwise."

ME: I know you meant well, but those gifts make me feel like you think I need fixing.

SCOTT: Oh, sorry! I wasn't fixing you, just helping you.

ME: I didn't think I needed help... Help with what?

SCOTT: Just with life. Everyone needs help sometimes.

ME: You seem like a really responsible guy, what with your bustling medicine cabinet and your two alarm clocks, but I don't want anybody thinking they're responsible for me. So if I'm not drowning or on fire, give me space and know that I can handle myself.

SCOTT: Oh. You seem very guarded. You know what would
help with that?

ME: Don't even!

As far as first arguments go, it was pretty civilized. We
agreed I'd drop better hints next February and he'd fix the
rest of the world except me. And he did. He's a magnet for
people who sweat all sizes of stuff, and for years had coun-
selled friends and even strangers through their tough times,
to the point that he eventually got proper certification and
hung out a shingle for Energy Healing and Spiritual Guid-
ance. But I had always resented the fairy-tale notion of a man
rescuing his lady from anything, be it dragon, poison, or the
sweating of tiny things, so I rejected the "helpful" health
magazine subscription he got me for my birthday, the "helpful" reminders to floss more than once a month, and the
one time he asked the most forbidden "helpful" question of
all: "Do you really need a third slice of cake?" In his defence,
his family shows love by worrying about each other. If one
doesn't dramatically exclaim, "Why are you eating so many
peanuts? You're gonna have a heart attack" in true Estelle
Costanza–style, then it's presumed you have no heart. But
he is a good listener, and eventually I convinced him that
even though his help is meant as kindness, it suffocates me,
so he stopped.

Fourteen years later, help with little things like cake or
floss or ill-timed literary gifts wouldn't have made a difference
anyway. I needed a full-on intervention. I was half-relieved
when after years of leaving me to my own miserable devices,
he put his foot down and insisted on fixing *us*. I agreed to, ugh,
see a marriage counsellor.

Scott googled "marriage" and "therapy" and "cheap" and presented me with several options. I was skeptical because I'd sought counselling before and it always came with a side order of awkwardness. One therapist fell asleep most sessions, one didn't shoo his dog away when it repeatedly humped my purse, and one just kept asking about the biz.

ME: I get a little gloomy every Janua—
PSYCHIATRIST: Yes, winter can be difficult. Seasonal affective disorder is very real. Are you working with anyone famous this winter?
ME: Uh, no.
PSYCHIATRIST: Are celebrities shorter in person? Have you ever met Tom Cruise, for example? I don't see him as being any tinier than he looks onscreen.

Seeing them left me only slightly less frazzled than before I'd made the appointment, so leading up to sofa-gate I was only under the care of my family doctor, a fun father figure who looked like Santa and had the velvety voice of Bob Barker.

ME: I still feel "off."
BEST DOCTOR: Listen, missy, you've GOT to see a psychiatrist.
ME: Right. I will.
BEST DOCTOR: (*pause*) I know a lie when I hear one.
ME: Heh-heh. You got me there. I wasn't really going to see a psychiatrist.
BEST DOCTOR: But you'll make an appointment this time?
ME: Sure.
BEST DOCTOR: You, missy, are a real pain.

He wrote referrals and made recommendations and I'd toss them out, still grateful for the twenty minutes we had to chat.

I visited him from the time my kids were born until he got sick and stopped working. I couldn't imagine finding anyone nearly as easygoing or understanding, so I went without a GP for a few years. I didn't feel like changing out of my pyjamas, never mind choosing someone potentially annoying to chart the course of my mental health. But, still, I owed it to Scott to at least consider the list of marriage counsellors he had emailed me from the other room.

That one's too far a drive...

Too many degrees—can't commit, probably flaky...

Ew, he's got a moustache—who does that?!

I huffily jimmied my phone back between the sofa cushions and shouted toward the door, "Just pick whoever's closest to Tim Hortons!"

I woke up the day of our first appointment feeling relieved to be handing the reins over to anyone other than ourselves. Scott and I took separate cars, even though we'd left the house at the same time, and nodded to each other like co-workers when we walked up to the therapist's house.

Please let this be the place that allows me to stop
ending every day with an apology.

We shuffled in quietly, as though entering a church mid-mass, and any skepticism I might have had faded when we got to the waiting room of her basement office: no margarine tubs of tiny half-dead plants, no spacey New Age music, none of that obnoxious "live, laugh, love, linger, leprechaun, etc." art—good start!

The therapist—let's call her Evelyn—looked like the kind of cozy, patient woman who could spend six hours silently hand-stitching a quilt. She was so still in her chair she might as well have been having her portrait painted. In fact, she had a bit of a *Mona Lisa* smile (with a Judge Judy hairdo).

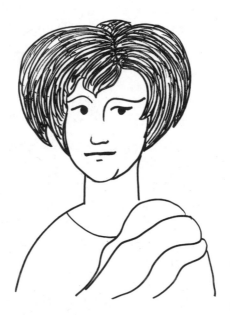

Her calmness was contagious, and Scott and I were yawning within minutes of sitting down. Being in such neutral territory, everything in me unwound, like when some nurse gives you a lice check in third grade, and even though you dread hearing a negative outcome, the effects of a two-minute scalp massage are well worth it. Or is that just me?

PAT: (*pause*) Uh...
ME: Moving on then!

After the usual intake questions of "Any drinkers in the family?" and "How did it make you feel when your brother was better at arm wrestling than you?" we got down to brass tacks. But just as I was prepping to unload the metaphorical Mack Truck of evidence I'd been compiling against Scott, I caught the innocent expression on his face. He looked tired, but also hopeful. For a moment I saw him as he was in our framed wedding photo: the perfect gentleman I kept in stitches. He's the guy who whispered "I'll do the dishes for the rest of your life" as an oddly charming sort of thank-you in the delivery room after our daughter was born (he kept that promise), who makes hilarious sound effects to pass the time when we're stuck in traffic, who ignores everyone's eye rolls as he tirelessly performs Reiki on our old, scrawny cat so she'll feel better. Now here we were, a pair of sad, wet rags seeking a ceasefire. My frustration downgraded to desperation, and I prefaced every piece of evidence against him with "I know I'm partly responsible, and this isn't a judgment, but… " I might have viewed him as the enemy, but I still loved the guy.

ME: Can we fix this?
EVELYN: We'll see.

We got up to leave so Evelyn could get back to (I assume) her quilting and I asked about scheduling our next appointment.

EVELYN: I'd like it if we could speak a little more openly. Would you please each come back and meet with me privately?

I did come back alone, and without the fear of wounding Scott more than I already had, I opened up.

EVELYN: So, I thought we'd start wi—

ME: Scott's the worst!!

EVELYN: Oh. Alright. What does he do exactly that bothers you?

ME: Everything. And I know most people use that term as an exaggeration, but I actually mean Every. Single. Thing.

EVELYN: Like?

ME: Like... he's this giant, cumbersome shape that's in the way. His huge shoes take up too much space. I'm always tripping over them. And he obsesses over being responsible and doing the right thing like a total keener! All I ask is that he handle everything so I can stop worrying about it, but instead he exhausts me. He's all like "Are you getting up today?" and "Aren't you gonna wipe that peanut butter off your chin? It's been there since yesterday." Enough already!

EVELYN: That must be hard for you. Does anyone else get under your skin?

ME: Uh, yes. A lot of people actually.

EVELYN: Your friends?

ME: Yeah. I just don't feel like they get me. And it's really draining being around them 'cause they always wanna hang out and have fun.

EVELYN: (*slight pause*) Mm-hmm. And what about your family?

ME: Super draining!

EVELYN: Your kids?

ME: Well, of course I like being with my kids. I'm not an arsehole! I mean, I'm kind of in a fog when I'm with them, but they're still my favourite people.

EVELYN: So you're foggy with your kids, and everyone else exhausts you?

ME: Uh, yeah. Yeah, that's accurate.

EVELYN: So it's not just Scott then.

ME: Well, no, I guess not. Hey, do you quilt, by chance?

EVELYN: Stick with me here, Jessica. You're saying you don't want to be around anyone anymore, except for your children, with whom you're foggy?

ME: Yeah. Is that not normal?

EVELYN: Well, it's normal in a depression.

ME: Oh come on! Am I depressed again?

EVELYN: (*sympathetic shrug*)

I was depressed, and that was the problem, not telemarketers, online shopping, people in general, the comedy industry at large, and Scott's big shoes, as I had originally hypothesized.

I enjoyed a moment's relief at the thought that my husband and I had hope.

It's just a temporary depression.

I don't have to be alone forever.

I can enjoy my life again someday.

I went through half a box of tissue, bawling out of relief that I might become close to my dish-doing husband again.

EVELYN: I'm referring you to a psychiatrist.

ME: Ok. And once the shrink fixes my noggin, we'll come back and make Scott more how I want him to be.

EVELYN: Oh. I wouldn't have used *any* of that vernacular, but, yes, I'm here if you need me.

My new psychiatrist—let's call her Dr. Huh 'cause "huh" was her catchphrase—was a no-nonsense academic type from somewhere in Great Britain who had neither a humpy dog, nor a fixation with celebrities, nor narcolepsy, so I was really impressed with her. It took her six seconds to confirm Evelyn's theory:

ME: So that's me in a nutshe—
DR. HUH: Huh, classic depression!

Getting a diagnosis is good because

a. I had an actual name and suggested course of treatment for what was wrong;
b. I finally had an excuse for my slothfulness: "Sorry I haven't cut the front lawn in two years. I'm depressed";
c. Scott realized I hadn't been body-snatched but was actually just on hiatus from my personality;
d. I could let my friends know why I'd been avoiding them for the last two years.

Getting a diagnosis is bad because

a. having a course of treatment at some point meant leaving the safety of my couch. And it's a really inviting couch. It's a velvet sectional for heaven's sake!
b. being depressed for a second time without obvious cause meant that I might be susceptible to reoccurrences. People who have suffered from more than one depression are considered in remission when they're better, not cured. To put it in poetic terms, it's the cold sore of the mind.

PAT: Gross!
ME: Precisely!

c. some people still don't believe depression is real, and may express that opinion subtly ("Oh, I'm sure you just need a little fresh air") or in a full Rodney Dangerfield impression:

"Depressed, eh? What, did the tooth fairy give you that diagnosis?" (*tie straighten*)

d. with any diagnosis comes advice. Depressed people loathe (Is there a stronger word than "loathe"? If so, insert that word here: _____) getting simplistic advice. Telling someone who feels like they're being crushed by an invisible elephant that "I've got this great acupuncturist you should try" or "my cousin eliminated wheat from his diet and his depression went away" is as effective as telling your cat, "From now on, chew with your mouth closed, ok?" It's well-intentioned, but it also implies that there's a fast fix for depression, like it's as elementary as following Ikea instructions:

SÄDSÄK

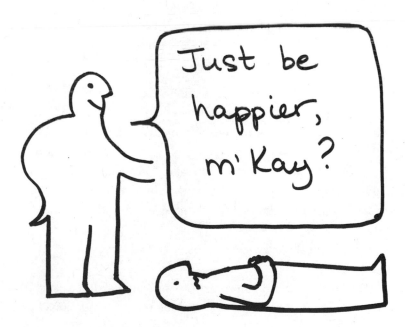

Advice just adds pressure to our hamster wheel of discouragement, and then we've gotta deal with the guilt of disappointing someone.

FRIEND: They say exercise releases endorphins.
ME: Yup.
FRIEND: So if you exercised more, you'd feel better.
ME: Uh-huh.
FRIEND: ... you should exercise.
ME: Yeah.
FRIEND: ... are you gonna do it? You know, exercise?
ME: No.
FRIEND: But it would make you feel better.
ME: Urmph.
FRIEND: Come on, it's so simple!
ME: Ugh! All this talking is exhausting. You should go. But first pass me that bag of corn chips I've been using as a footrest.
FRIEND: Ew, they expired six months ago.
ME: Stop judging me!!

If I could have waved a wand and made my friends the ultimate support tool, they would have had ESP to know exactly how bad I felt despite my lies and excuses, and dropped by often to binge-watch sophomoric TV with me, providing validation during commercial breaks: "Must be hard. Sorry, buddy." But I suppose that's what moms are for and that is exactly what mine did for a weekend every month.

I'm super lucky, for a person in a pool of despair.

Dr. Huh was a woman of action, and she used her psychiatric witchcraft to trick me into making recommendations for myself (only 66 percent of which I discarded immediately), as well as starting me on some antidepressants. The pharmacist explained that it could take six to eight weeks for the medication to have full effect.

PHARMACIST: You may experience nausea, dry mouth, and anxiety in the first few weeks, but that's standard and nothing to worry about.
ME: Ok. If I feel worried, I will not worry about it.

Getting a diagnosis *then* having to wait for the treatment to work is surreal—sort of like if a dog chomped down on your leg and the veterinarian says, "Classic case of dog-on-leg. Don't worry, we'll get him off in two months. Just hang tight and try to act natural."

In the meantime, Dr. Huh suggested Scott and I find a few things that we could rebond over. We tried to woo each other into our respective hobbies:

SCOTT: Wanna clean the house together? It'll give you a great feeling of accomplishment!
ME: No. Wanna binge-watch a reality series where husbands swap wives with each other for a week? It'll give you a great feeling of moral superiority.
SCOTT: That's awful. Wanna sit together and read?
ME: Ew! How about we surf Facebook and see who's doing better than us?
SCOTT: Wow, that's just... no.
ME: Would you consider going on a trip somewhere?
SCOTT: Hmmmm...

I love nature, but in the past Scott had avoided going out into the wilderness because "Jews don't camp." We came up with a compromise and booked a last-minute trip to Mexico with Genna's family so that we could reignite the fun times that attracted us to each other 'cause that's what does the trick in Adam Sandler rom coms (although in his movies they don't show the scene where Scott and I bicker about the expense even though I clearly explained, "But I have a prescription for fun times!"). Genna, Anson (he's the guy from the introduction who owns red *Magnum, P.I.* short-shorts, remember?), Scott, and the kids were thrilled to arrive at the resort; thrilled with the rooms, the pool, the ocean, the food. Me, I had a different reaction to paradise...

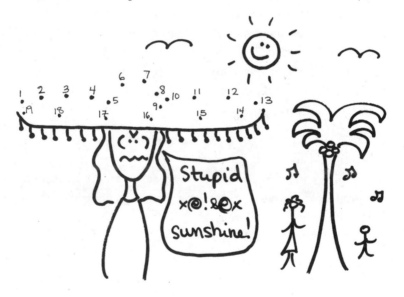

ME: Pat, did you connect the dots?
PAT: I didn't have to. It's clearly a somb—
ME: Shhh! Don't give it away!

Instead of finding my smile among friends and foliage, I immediately felt jealous of Genna. She has boundless energy and it was making me feel like a stick-in-the-mud in comparison. She and I used to be birds of a feather, and I mean that literally. I'd raised zebra finches as a kid, cartoonish little birds that beep instead of chirp, and ever since we'd met in third grade Genna and I would spontaneously beep at each other in private and public alike. Lately when she beeped at me, I'd just nod in acknowledgment. And now, while I was busy looking for things to complain about ("Honestly, does the sun have to be that g#%$^&mned bright?!"), she was whimsically twirling down the beach, flowers in her hair and a swing in her step. "Jessie, dance with me," she called. She was effervescent.

That used to be me.

I muttered "no" and wandered off to the bar to order "mucho rum with un poquito Coke, por favor."

PAT: Oh, were you supposed to mix alcohol with that medication?
ME: (*silence*)
PAT: I see.

Adding a booze-induced fog to my depressive fog didn't make me any more pleasant. Despite how hard I tried to be couple-y and vacation-y, annoyed was my go-to reaction, and it was as ingrained in me as telling someone "bless you" after a sneeze.

SCOTT: Hey luv, wanna try the lazy river with us?
ME: Seriously?! If you wanna float down a waterway of kid pee, knock yourself out!

The resort's "Kids Club" consisted of a bag of candy and some heavily goobered stuffed animals, so we kept the young 'uns with us. Despite a few choice moments, I spent most of the week woozily yelling "Don't drown!" and "Don't drink the lazy river water!" I was relieved when the trip was over, as there were no secluded sectionals with a clear view of the TV at this resort. And that, folks, is basically depression in a nutshell: the world is your oyster but you can't see past your own misery.

When we got back home, I told Dr. Huh about how I'd resigned myself to just be miserable "till the pills cure me," and that's when she explained that the pills may only be one small part of the equation, and not a cure-all.

DR. HUH: We need to take a multi-faceted approach.

ME: Ugh. You saying that makes me even more tired. Now I have to double my time on the sectional. But how?? There's only twenty-four hours in each day!

DR. HUH: Antidepressants may help people with severe depression, but studies go back and forth on whether they're effective in moderate or mild cases versus using a placebo. Do you know what a placebo is?

ME: Yes. It's when doctors give you a useless pill instead of the real McCoy to see if *thinking* you're being healed makes you feel better, and maybe also to laugh in private about how gullible you are.

DR. HUH: Huh. Your best chance at getting better involves more than just a prescription. After all, a painkiller may cure your headache, but that doesn't mean that headaches are caused by a shortage of painkillers.

ME: (*blank stare*)

DR. HUH: I'm saying you have work to do.

ME: Yuck.

Dr. Huh helped me differentiate which of our marital problems were superficial and easily worked on (not sharing a bathroom solves so many problems), and which ones would require a deeper psychological shift (acknowledging that the world was not, in fact, against me).

The superficial problems were fairly obvious. We both worked from home, and being in close quarters twenty-four hours a day was ... too much of a good thing, to put it politely.

PAT: Good spin.

ME: Thanks!

We tried to make our home office like a real one, although we didn't go as far as passing a card around "the office" for birthdays or punching a time card when we took a lunch break. Working from home is not all it's cracked up to be. It's like every day is casual Friday. And every lunch hour is potluck, but I'm the only one who brings anything, 'cause Scott always says, "Hey, can you just make twice as much of whatever you're bringing?" At the start you're like "all this freedom!" but then within a month you're not even bothering to get dressed in the morning—just wandering around in your PJs eating cereal right out of the box. When I saw Scott puttering around the house, it felt like he was holding up a mirror to how unproductive I was, regardless of the fact that puttering is just his natural state and he finds it meditative. Since our house is open concept, when Scott had clients, I'd reluctantly peel myself off the sofa and hide in the bedroom for an hour and a half watching Netflix on my phone with the volume turned down. If the kids were home they joined me, all three of us hunched over a four-inch screen, nibbling on snacks I was now storing in the dresser, straining to hear. I didn't want Scott's clients in my space, noticing my sloth-fulness, like that one guy who caught me skulking from the bedroom to the kitchen in my bathrobe to restock on pop-corn, and asked, "How you have a house? I no see you work!" Caught off guard, I answered truthfully, "I was real ambitious before I got depressed." As soon as he had enough clients, Scott moved his business to a small shared office nearby.

For a few hours each week I reached out to get our home and finances in shape. I asked my accountant to tally up what my online shopping habit was costing us annually.

ACCOUNTANT: In a nutshell, ouch.

We went on a budget, which is a term I use loosely. We finally got back the money we invested in that film (lesson learned), went down to one car, quit ordering fast food, and downgraded our debt from mountainous to hilly.

A friend of ours is a professional organizer, and after a walk-through she observed, "It seems like when you guys can't find something, instead of looking for two minutes, you go out and buy a replacement right away." Which explained why we had duplicate staplers, ironing boards, and artifi-cial Christmas trees. It also explained why visitors often remarked, "Oh, are you moving or something?" when they saw boxes of stuff piled everywhere. We sent over thirty garbage bags of goods to a thrift store, and even some bags of less-than-goods (like mismatched socks and a tangle of incompatible electrical cords from the '90s) until the guy at the drop-off door remarked, "You know we're not a garbage can, right?" I still had plenty of work to do on an individual level, but at least Scott and I had shooed out a few of the ele-phants in the room.

The following spring, work had picked up some, so we cashed in all our travel miles and joined Genna for her fortieth birthday in Hawaii. She was renting a house on the island of Kauai, just a few blocks from Poipu Beach. We packed some snacks and fruity cocktails and headed to the waterfront for a day of lazing in the sun (well, her in the sun, me hiding under a large umbrella in my full length UPF 50+ swimwear). After an hour I realized sunbathing in the shade is really just napping, so I put on a mask and snorkel and walked into the water. The reef started a few feet from the water's edge, and within minutes I saw a rainbow of coral and fish. I floated around, taking it all in. I'd seen reefs this diverse on TV, but never in person. When some waves slammed me into a shallow patch of rough coral and I had to flail embarrassingly to free myself, I only winced a little instead of shouting "the world is against me" and going home to cry in bed for the rest of the day.

That was odd. Have the pills finally kicked in?

I hadn't noticed a difference in the seven months since I'd started taking them, but I wondered if maybe this reasonable human-like reaction was a start. The next day Genna took us to a hiking trail she'd heard about, which I later learned fell under the description of "treacherous and dangerous" in the guidebooks. It took seven hours and I ran out of water in the first thirty minutes. It was a terrifying climb and when we reached a crumbling cliff that was barely attached to the mountain, I thought of my children and we turned back. Genna did not think of her children and she kept going. Moments after we separated from the group, Scott twisted his ankle, and we had to walk backwards down the mountain, one step at a time, with him leaning his giant frame on me for support. When we reached the bottom, we sat down on a log.

SCOTT: I know that wasn't easy for you. Thanks for keeping your cool.
ME: Yeah, that was weird, huh?

I was extremely thirsty, but the idiot in me thought that only sissies drink water on vacation so I kept boozing it up until dinner, when I switched to wine, "which is basically water before Jesus gets a hold of it." The waiter told us, "Just keep looking over the horizon at the sunset. Eventually you'll see a whale." I didn't see a whale, but after thirty minutes of staring at the sun, I did get photo-flash vision distortion (known as an "aura") leading right into a migraine. Scott guided me back to our room, put a cool cloth on my head, and gave me painkillers from the first aid travel kit I had jibed him for packing two days earlier. At 2 a.m. I woke up and started vomiting uncontrollably, and when it didn't subside after fifteen ralphs, I made miming motions to Scott to call 9-1-1. An ambulance took me to the hospital, where I was treated for dehydration, only checking out the next afternoon when it was time to fly home. A sudden flurry of panic hit me.

ME: How much does the hospital cost?! Isn't it, like, $10,000 a day for an American hospital?? I'm gonna have to sell a kidney—both kidneys!
SCOTT: It's ok. I got insurance. They took care of everything.
ME: Oh. (*pause*) That was smart of you.

I leaned into him.

ME: I don't like Hawaii.
SCOTT: Me either.

And we stayed together like a pair of Velcro-armed monkeys for five minutes, which is longer than the sum total of our hugs in the previous two years.

PAT: But, Jess, did Scott use the hall pass you mentioned in the last chapter?
ME: Oh, I forgot about that. I never asked him, so who knows.
PAT: Why didn't you ask him?
ME: (*loud sigh*) Because I think he should have done whatever he needed to get through the nightmare, short of murdering me. It's time to forgive and forget and all that junk.
PAT: Can you go ask him now?
ME: No!

Sometimes, when we're doing nothing in particular, we'll bond over how much we hate Hawaii, while Genna shakes her head at us. It reminds me that in all of my worst moments, Scott has been there, holding up my proverbial hair so the proverbial puke doesn't get on it. And that's love. That's marathon-worthy.

Humiliation Fee

. . . . .

I NEVER FELT like I was a comedian's comedian, 'cause I'm a morning person and I don't smoke pot. In fact, since most of what I do are private shows for corporations, it's possible other comedians are completely unaware that I am a comedian, too. Like when a baby mouse who's been handled by a human is returned to the litter, the other mice reject it for not smelling 100 percent mousy and get all "What are you, an ox? You don't smell right! Mom's gonna eat you!" I fly so far under the radar that when I ran into a casting director last year, she asked, "You're a real estate agent now, right?" I'd like to think she just made the assumption because I have the jazzy polish of a realtor:

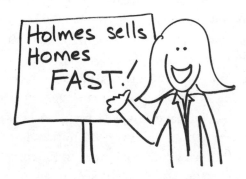

...and not because I've entirely disappeared from the comedy community. But there's a reason I relocated in the Comedian Protection Program: I found my peers intimidating (even more than the icy, sexy people at the gym who wear muscle shirts and pay for extra oxygen in their water). Maybe my fearfulness stemmed from the culture shock of going from modest Mormon to beer-hall clown, or insecurity about my material being less joke-based and more character-based than theirs, or from an incident at the start of my career when I was recording my performance on a tape recorder placed in the green room and the next morning when I listened to the tape, I discovered the recording had picked up other comedians mocking me backstage.

PAT: Oh, that's awful. Like, I wanna throw up.
ME: Wait, there's more!

At one of my first open mic nights, the emcee was whipping a rubber chicken at any performer who wasn't getting enough laughs—while they were still on stage!! The flogged amateurs skulked away as the emcee merrily picked up the chicken and introduced the next potential target. I didn't get hit with the chicken but I felt so anxious I might as well have been. I was in awe of comedians individually—so quick and daring and brave. I was inspired by them when we hung out solo, but in a group setting, the one-upmanship made me anxious, and to quote Michael Jackson quoting someone else, "I'm a lover, not a fighter." I withdrew from the social side of my job, going against the expression "don't throw out the baby with the bathwater" (which, by the way, is surely the worst expression ever, and we need to find an equivalent— maybe "don't throw out the remote with the recycling." Meh, I'll keep working on it) and mostly kept to myself at the clubs.

Years later I'd become so far removed from my comedy peers that I didn't turn to them when I needed support for what many in our industry go through—tough crowds, dry spells, depressions, humiliations.

Ahhhh, the humiliations.

No matter how successful you are, everybody has a price for which they'll do something they know is artistically a terrible call:

- Cher's repetitive hair infomercials went on to be mercilessly mocked on *SNL*, which I can only assume is what led to her singing, "If I could turn back ta-ham!"
- Rob Lowe was midway through a cringe-worthy duet with Snow White at the 1989 Academy Awards when he looked into the audience and saw director Barry Levinson mouthing the words, *What the f#$k?*
- Bill Murray did *Garfield* because he was a big fan of the writer/director Joel Coen, who, he was told, had written the script. When he showed up to voice Garfield and didn't like the script, he realized the movie was written by Joel Cohen, the guy who directed *Monster Mash: The Movie*, and not Joel Coen, the guy who co-wrote and directed *Fargo*. What a difference an "h" makes!
- George Clooney kept a photo of himself as Batman, complete with pointy plastic nipples, on his office wall for years as a cautionary reminder not to make bad movies solely for the money.
- It took Roseanne Barr years to recover from her disastrous singing of the national anthem at a Padres game where 50,000 fans booed, threw beer bottles, and fat-shamed her. President Bush himself publicly reprimanded her.
- When Halle Berry showed up in person to collect her Razzie for "Worst Performance by a Female" in *Catwoman*,

she thanked the studio for "putting me in that piece of sh*t." And THAT, my friends, is the only way to come out of a humiliation with your head held high!

In the sterile world of corporate comedy, we experience the odd humiliation, too. Not just the expected challenge of a tough crowd, but the manoeuvring required to get over a bad set-up. When you're hired to do stand-up, you expect a) a stage, b) a microphone, and c) an audience seated in an enclosed space. I am amazed how many shows I've been booked on that not only didn't have at least one or two of those factors, but also had extra challenges thrown in. I affectionately call some cheques "humiliation fees," when my contract contains any combination of the following red flags:

- Carnival
- Kids
- Birthday party
- Poolside
- Outdoors
- Enter stage coming down a three-storey slide
- Live bear will be at side of the stage during some of her performance

I said yes to every one of those gigs (fortunately the bear was a no-show) because I was a starving artist for so long that it became ingrained in me that any gig, even an obstacle-rich one (see how I spun that?), beats no gig at all.

AGENT: You probably want to pass on this one. They have you performing in a cavernous, circular atrium, and they've asked that you lean slightly over the balcony for the entirety of your performance so the whole audience five storeys down can see you.

ME: Sign me up!

AGENT: Jess, I really wouldn't do this one—the pay is peanuts, there'll be a terrible echo for sound, and I'd be concerned for your safety.

ME: Hmm. Do they validate parking?

AGENT: Yes. But you're successful now, so you don't need to take—

ME: I'm in!

That particular gig was as bad as you'd imagine, not just for me bent over a balcony shouting, but for the two hundred employees down below craning their necks and wincing at the sound of a squawking Liza Minnelli impression bouncing off marble walls. But it's a bit like going on a terrifying roller coaster: when you're at the crest of a gargantuan hill you think, "Wait, why would I do this? This is the worst possible choice I could have made." Then later, when things are a little too still and settled, you miss the rush, and you reconsider.

Being terrified has its perks!

Having your ego inflated then deflated comes with the job: I opened for Jerry Seinfeld one night, and the next night bombed at a poolside comedy show where precocious (that's the nice word for "arsehole") kids splashed me throughout my set. If I were to exclaim, "I'm shocked by that dud audience," I'd have my comedy licence revoked (well, I'd remind the comedy club I'm a member and THEN they'd revoke it).

Sometimes the humiliation is self-inflicted, like when I wore six-inch stilettos on stage to give me great confidence but the heels of my shoes kept poking through the grates in the makeshift stage, leaving me no choice but to remove the shoes and do the show barefoot (and with little confidence, but GREAT comfort). Or when my bangs got stuck to the glue of my false eyelashes and I couldn't blink for a fifteen-minute routine emceeing for Russell Peters.

Other times it's an oversight: I was hired to perform at a remote corporate event with no green room or backstage area. The organizer wanted me to be a surprise so they asked me to hide in a bathroom for three hours. I ate a vending machine dinner on the cold porcelain seat, standing every ten minutes so my legs wouldn't fall asleep.

And sometimes—often, actually—you don't get the whole story upfront. For example, once I had paid my dues and gotten some starring roles on TV, someone hired me to play Martha Stewart at an upscale party.

ME: Oh, I actually don't do a very good Martha. Is there someone else I can do a parody of? Britney Spears? Michael Jackson?

CLIENT: It's all settled. Everyone's going to love your Martha!

I showed up to the party dressed in a blond bob wig and understated cardigan and khakis. I found the organizer and asked, "So where will I be performing?" She handed me a cheese tray and said, "Just go be Martha offering everyone cheese. Do a bit of a show for each person." I've heard of up-close magic—in fact a friend of mine does it at restaurants, walking from table to table performing tricks, er, I mean *illusions*, for people. But up-close comedy? I turned again to the organizer to protest, but she enthusiastically waved me forward, like "Go accept your Academy Award!" I went from person to person, and with a droll flare and deep voice said, "You'll want to try the cheese. It's from the Nubian goats on my Connecticut farm. I milked them myself. It's a good thing." It became clear very quickly that no one had been told a comedian would be part of the evening's entertainment, because everyone awkwardly averted their gaze when I started my spiel, or they'd grab a cheese hunk and walk away while I was mid-monologue. To them I was not an entertainer, but a haughty weirdo with a dairy fetish. People handed me their soiled napkins, asked where the washrooms were, and told me they needed their wine topped up. "I'll let the kitchen know," I replied.

Would I do it again? Yes. Because… money. As someone who used to sell garbage bags door to door for four bucks an hour, I've done worse for less. And because I really do love my job, even when the circumstances are less than optimal/ verging on absurd. There's usually a moment of deep fulfillment on stage, when creativity is flowing through me and I feel the audience's laughter right in my core. I give them the best version of

Jessica Holmes

I can, connecting in a way I can't (or don't) in my offstage, introverted life as jessica holmes.

Even after Seinfeld had his success on, well, *Seinfeld*, he went back and started over in small comedy clubs, trying out new material. In the documentary *Comedian*, when he was asked about returning to this kind of reverse-dues-paying, he replied, "One day I was watching these construction workers go back to work. Just watching them trudging down the street. It was just like a revelation to me. I realized, 'These guys don't wanna go back to work after lunch. But they're going. 'Cause that's their job.' And if they can exhibit *that* level of dedication for *that* job, I should be able to do the same. Just trudge your ass in."

It's an honour to work in comedy. Who am I to turn down a gig?

PAT: But bombing must take its toll.

ME: Oh for sure. Of course. But I've been on stage for twenty years, so while it's still an awful feeling, I can look at it objectively. Like I'd been shown a chart in advance that explains the science of live comedy and how if you're having an off night or performing at an outdoor medieval festival, competing with drunken passersby dressed like witches or wenches or knights in full armour (and Nikes), you're mathematically less likely to get a standing ovation. The logic takes some of the sting out.

PAT: Unless you're Kevin Hart. Now he's funny anywh—

ME: Don't you dare, Pat. Don't you dare play the Kevin Hart card!

PAT: Heh-heh. Ok.

But when I was depressed, and completely lacking resilience, it was a whole other story. Logic and math and rational thinking didn't apply. A common symptom of depression is not being able to fathom a time when you won't feel as down as you currently do. It's like you become emotionally nearsighted. If I bombed when I was depressed, I went from "That was a bad gig" to "I'm untalented and we'll be living in our RV within a year." It also makes you withdraw from the very peers whose support you need most. So not only are you sad, you are sad *and* alone with these problems. The most isolating belief I had when I was depressed was that I was the only person with this pain. Identifying with someone else in your situation is one of the hardest, but most important, things a depressed person can do.

Part of recovering was reaching out more to my peers and asking, "Hey, do you go through what I go through?" I'd clicked with wonderful people at Second City and in the comedy circuit through the years, but I kept my distance because of a few bad experiences and never got to a place where I thought of comedians as "my people." But now I had to push past that limiting belief for the sake of my mental health. Coming out of depression can be freeing, in that you've already hit what feels like rock bottom, and you wonder, "What else is there to lose if I just be myself and be honest and open?"

I was in the green room at Ottawa's Cracking-up the Capital festival (an event that raises money and awareness for mental illness through comedy) last spring and decided to reach out to the emcee, Patrick McKenna (*The Red Green Show*, *Remedy*), who has been open about his struggles with mental health. I told him, "For the most part, my life is great. But when I have a tough gig, it casts a shadow over everything else and makes me feel like a fraud." He nodded understandingly and told me about corporate comedians who bomb more often than they succeed and who are still considered extremely successful. "Sometimes it's how the gigs are set up. They want someone funny on the bill to create some buzz leading up to the event, but when it comes to the actual show, they don't worry whether anyone listens. They're busy networking." The scrunched-up knots in my shoulders loosened.

It's not just me. My problems are not unique.

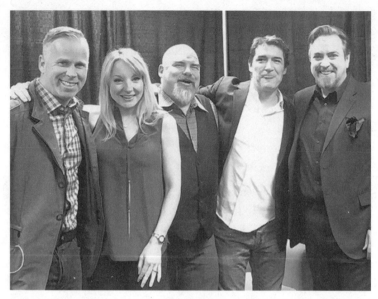

In the Cracking-up the Capital green room with comedians Gerry Dee, Tazz Norris, Tim Steeves, and Patrick McKenna. Photo courtesy of Scott McMann.

Tazz Norris, a successful stand-up, overheard us and piped in, "We're all here for each other. Just reach out whenever you need a reminder that you're not alone."

Those fellas were so convincing that I decided to work in a group setting more often—accepting a gig in a writers' room, performing with other improvisers at fundraisers, returning to *Royal Canadian Air Farce* for annual TV specials. The bullies were fewer and farther between than I remembered. I pushed past the voice in my head that told me "they don't consider you their peer" and shamelessly asked folks to share their cringe-worthy stories for this book. I'm happy to report they didn't get all "you don't smell right" as I hypothesized at the beginning of the chapter. Instead, they readily shared their most humiliating adventures in comedy with me. I picked my favourites. Enjoy, Pat!

PAT: I will—thanks!

SFX: '80s game show music

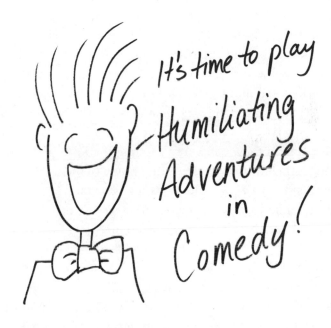

PAT: Is that your husband? The game show host?

ME: Sure is! Thanks, Scott.

SCOTT: No problem. Am I needed for the rest of the chapter, or was it just that opening line? 'Cause I was gonna make a sandwich.

ME: You're all good. I can take it from here. (*Ahem*) Here are tonight's—

SCOTT: Hi again, sorry, Jess did you want a sandwich?

ME: No thanks.

SCOTT: Pat?

PAT: Uh, no thanks. I'm not even sure how that would work.

ME: We're good, Scotty. (*Ahem*) Here are tonight's finalists!

Bad Pre-show Intel

James Cunningham, a seasoned stand-up and TV personality, likes to riff on the fact that he is bald. He even asks clients in advance to give him the name of a good-natured bald man in the audience. On one such occasion he was given a man's name (let's call him Carl). James launched into his comedy, slinging one zinger after another about Carl's baldness, and wondering why the audience stared, open-mouthed, at him. James figured they just weren't *getting* the joke, and zinged stronger than before, really hitting home the fact that Carl's baldness is what we should all be focusing on. He found out after the show that Carl has alopecia, a disease that limits hair growth. To quote James, "They hated me."

They Don't Get the Joke

Comedian Simon B. Cotter, who is hilarious, was asked to roast a very prestigious doctor who was retiring. All of the doctor's peers gathered to see Simon pay tribute to their colleague. The doctor's first delivery forty years earlier was a baby born in a train car. Simon, hoping to customize his set, made a joke that HE was that baby delivered by the doctor forty years earlier, and he made up stories about what a fantastical life he had lived thanks to the doctor's handy delivery-work. Though the audience was laughing at Simon's made-up story, the old doctor somehow missed the joke and got up and gave a tear-filled speech about how much that event had influenced his practice of medicine and how he had always wondered what happened to that baby, "who now stands before me as a man." All this while a room full of people stared at Simon, now with hatred, for (seemingly) tricking and humiliating a kind old doctor. Simon left without asking for his cheque.

Someone Thinks They Own You Because They Bought a Ticket to Your Show

Second City-favourite Jennifer Irwin was paying her dues acting in murder mystery dinner theatre. The gig barely paid, but she got to eat a free steak dinner during her shift. The hitch was she had only fifteen minutes to eat it, in full character, sitting with the guests. "There was always one a**hole who was determined to get his money's worth," she says. One night a man kept interrupting her meal and taunting her. She politely explained—in character—"I must eat to keep up my strength and solve this most complicated murder," and he replied, "Well, if you spent more time working on your acting and less time reaching for the Heinz, you might actually make a career out of show business." She didn't retaliate because she needed the job, so she ate silently while he proceeded to make fat jokes. She has gone on to star in the series *Still Standing*, *Eastbound & Down*, and *The Goldbergs*. Betcha she eats steak any time she likes.

They Literally Want Toilet Humour

Stand-up and radio host Dean Young was hired for a kids' comedy-themed bar mitzvah. His job was to stand in the restroom at the Ritz Carlton in downtown Toronto and heckle guys while they came in and used the facilities. For four hours he roasted anyone who came in to do their business. He could hear the DJ continuously announcing the disclaimer, "There is a grown man in the men's lavatory speaking to kids."

ME: Thanks for sharing, guys.
ALL COMEDIANS: Our pleasure. See how nice we are?
ME: Yes! I really do!

Nothing is as big a relief as having even one person validate your feelings; commiserating about humiliations or obstacles, big or small. My favourite words are "I've been there, buddy." Maybe for you comedy isn't the trigger. Maybe it's your relatives or a horrible boss or, like, say you work at a bank and people keep bringing in those giant six-foot-wide cheques or twirling their moustache and peering at you through their monocle; the answer—

PAT: Uh, do you go to many banks? 'Cause it sounds like you're just describing the rich guy from Monopoly?
ME: Yeah, I gotta get out more!

—the answer will still be the same. Even if you're too guarded, busy, shy, etc., getting validation makes a huge difference. Now, when I'm asked to work the term "S&P/TSX Composite Index" into a joke, or when I realize my stage is actually a fridge on its side, or when I'm shouting jokes at a room of 500 people because someone forgot to rent a mic, I think, "Wait till so-and-so hears about this—we'll have an *epic* laugh!"

Invent the Invisibility Cloak Already!

· · · · ·

MY NAME IS Jessica and I'm scared of people.

Phew. There. It's out in the open now. Introversion addressed! What my friends have long suspected about me—the eye rolls when I leave a dinner party at 8 p.m. or hide in the basement like a fugitive when the doorbell rings; the disappointment when I say, "I'm just going to the ladies' room," but then I slip out the back door of the bar—it's true: I'm a lone wolf. A lone wolf with a very public job.

For an introvert like me, it helps that people in Toronto are too busy or too rude to talk to each other. There's an unspoken rule that you can pretend to be alone in a big group. You look around on a crowded subway and realize everyone's in their own little bubble of solitude, reading a book or falling asleep with their mouth open or picking at their nails like no one else was around. Neighbours understand if you come out the front door of the house you can't afford with your head down, typing away on your phone, and ignore them as you race to your car. We're always stressed out because 90 percent of our paycheque goes to the mortgage (yet we're still wasting our remaining dollars on artisanal dog treats and organic hipster food that's supposed to be cooked, but you pay twice as much for it 'cause they serve it raw. I suppose one could just eat out of the neighbour's compost bin and save $80).

My point is, I'm most comfortable being squished together and simultaneously left alone. I do love people, just indirectly. To quote Marlin in *Finding Nemo*: "It's because I like you, I don't want to be with you. It's a very complicated emotion." One of my favourite things to do is have half a dozen friends over and *not* talk to them—just eavesdrop on all of their conversations while I cook dinner. Everyone saunters over to ask "Can I help?" and I say, "No thanks. Just keep chatting with each other," like someone who doesn't want their favourite TV show interrupted. They're used to it by now. Even when we're hanging together in one of their backyards, no one bats an eyelash when I pull a lounge chair into their circle, plunk my hat over my face, and pretend to be asleep while I quietly enjoy their company, piping up only when a punchline is needed.

It started as an assertiveness thing—panic in the face of confrontation. I can hold my own in front of thousands of people, but I become world-record-holdingly awkward if I have to tell one person that they gave me the wrong change. My fight-or-flight response thinks a difference of opinions is the same as being attacked by a bear. For this reason, I made a terrible roommate. The fridge alone was a minefield of confrontation: you set rules that this shelf is yours, and this shelf is mine, but condiments are a no man's land. Someone uses the last of my margarine and I screw up my attempt to handle it casually:

ME: Listen, why? (*deep breath*) It's just . . . who ate margarine's gone?

ROOMMATE: Huh? I ran out of butter so I used that other stuff.

ME: I can't believe you couldn't believe it's not butter!

ROOMMATE: Honest mistake. Chill out, dude. (*It was the early '90s.*)

ME: I am chilled out. My hands always shake like this. And, too, your clothes always stay in the dryer long after they're dry. It's a dryer, not a dresser, right? (*cough*) Just saying. Just chilling.

ROOMMATE: It looks like you're choking on air.

ME: I'll start looking for a new place.

Of course, I could have just said, "Hey, do you mind replacing the margarine if you use mine up?" but since assertiveness wasn't one of my basic life skills, I wouldn't have gotten through the sentence without developing a face rash, choking on my own spit, and yelling "nevermind!" too loudly while running out of the room. So my subsequent university years were spent in a tiny cockroach-infested bachelor pad where a guy down the hall repeatedly tried to sell me knives and sex trade workers conducted business below my window while I folded a pillow over my ears. I thought that was better than having a roommate.

After years of me self-diagnosing as "just weird," my friend Cara did a Myers-Briggs personality test on me and declared, "Oh, you're an introvert. That's what's been wrong with y—I mean, been going on this whole time!" And I felt like I had just discovered my true identity. I only have a few "people hours" in me per day. They're fun, boisterous, bonding hours. But when the people hours are used up, I have to close up shop or else I'll pay for all my hoopla the next day by feeling anxious and withdrawn. It's like eating: once you've burned up all your calories, you have to eat again otherwise you will crash. Units of alone time are my calories, and I burn out if I don't get them. Whether or not my friends understand it, they lovingly pretend it doesn't faze them when I say, "Pick dinner OR a movie 'cause I can't handle both."

PAT: It sounds like you have a lot of friends, you know, for a...

ME: For a weirdo? Yeah, I seem to have tapped into a very patient group. Plus I glom on to Genna's friends. She's the most patient of them all.

GENNA: I sure am!

ME: Genna! When did you get here??

GENNA: Just a second ago. Wanted to see if you're up for coffee today?

ME: No thanks. I already took a conference call, then the neighbour caught me sneaking from the car to the house, and then it was all "You know, if your lawn mower's broken you can always borrow mine" and I had to explain that our mower's not broken, we've just had a busy three months, so...

GENNA: Burned up your people hours early in the day, huh? No problemo. I'll try you again tomorrow.

ME: Cool. (*impersonating a zebra finch*) Beep beep.

GENNA: Beep beep.

BOTH: Beep b-beep b-beep beep.

GENNA: See ya.

PAT: Wow. Unreal.

ME: Yeah, she's a keeper!

I've looked for coping mechanisms for my introversion, including coming up with a list of conversation-enders if I've already spent my people hours. I'm partial to replying "I hear ya" or "Anything's possible" to most small talk. Just letting it hang there...

STRANGER: It's so cold out today.
ME: I hear ya. Anything's possible.
STRANGER: Well, uh, what?

Cab rides are tricky. If you answer one question, you set a precedent for having to chat the whole ride. Sometimes "anything's possible" isn't enough and you just have to resort to lying.

ME: Can I please go to Yonge and Bloor?
CABBIE: Sure. You have business there?
ME: Anything's possible.
CABBIE: Anything IS possible! That's why I came to this country. Now my children are going to university here! What is your line of work?
ME: ... data entry.
CABBIE: What kind of data?
ME: Whatever my boss gives me. Usually numbers.
THEM: Sounds vague.
ME: I hear ya.
CABBIE: Haven't I seen you on TV?
ME: Ummmmm. Not sure.
CABBIE: Yes. Yes, you're that girl who does the funny voices. Why are you doing data entry? Are you suffering a career setback and having to supplement your income?
ME: Please just let me off here.
CABBIE: We're twenty blocks away. This is a very dangerous neighbourhood.
ME: Anything's possible.

I was on set with a certain established actor (it was Gene Hackman!) who wore headphones when we weren't film-ing. "Oh," I thought, "what's he listening to?" I snuck close enough to see his Walkman (still the '90s) and noticed it was turned off. Dude was passively enjoying some downtime! On lone-wolf days, when I'm completely out of people hours, I've tried the headphone ruse, even wearing the giant puffy kind when I leave the house for a jog, but it doesn't work for me like it does for Gene. Some friendly dog walker will saunter in front of me and make small talk (including one eccentric gal who speaks to me in the loud made-up voices of her dogs, which I would normally consider a hoot but not when I'm hanging on by a thread. On those days her Scooby-Doo-esque "prease ron't run raway!" feels oppressive). If only I were ballsy enough to make myself a shirt that explained my predicament.

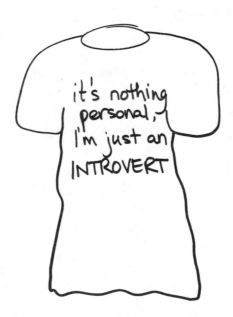

Then I could just jog by while they read me.

For airports and long flights, I'd give anything for an invisibility cloak. I saw them for sale on Etsy! They're working out the kinks, I guess (the disclaimer says "not an actual invisibility cloak"). Soon we'll be able to hide in plain sight willy-nilly à la Harry Potter, eavesdrop on a conversation, or just sneak into our parents' house and throw our laundry in with theirs. But that's not what I want the cloak for. I've just had a lot of moments when I'd like to be magically swallowed whole and disappear.

So far what I'm describing is just extreme introversion. There are books and cats to help with that. I am "special" and have an added complication: while I rarely get stage fright, I do suffer from social anxiety the day or two leading up to a show. And sometimes when I travel. Or when I'm a guest at someone else's house or when someone wants me to watch their kids or when I'm the "celebrity" grand marshal at a parade in Ottawa where I'm told to wave non-stop at people who keep shrugging at each other like "I don't know who she is?!" I hyper-worry that I can't meet the social expectations strangers have of me and it leaves me short of breath, anxious, and sometimes on the blue sofa for twenty-four hours. Pre-show, my behaviour vacillates between catatonic and scattered in a way that might make a psychiatrist say, "I'm going to forgo all medical terminology and simply call this behaviour what it is: spaz-like." When my social anxiety was at its worst and my depression was looming, I googled whether it was offensive to wear a burka on days when I wasn't up to chatting with strangers. Google said it was a jerk move. Regardless, I bailed on the plan when a friend pointed out that some cabbies might speak Farsi and I'd be found out in no time anyway. Nope, there was no beating this anxiety except chemically.

PAT: Actually, there are plenty of ways. You could try meditation, visualization, breathing techniques...
ME: Sounds awful!

My therapist prescribed me a drug that treats agitation
and anxiety. Within weeks it made me feel comfortable
under most circumstances, even when comfortable wasn't the
appropriate response. Like, whatever my question was, my
brain answered with a smooth Kate-Hudson-on-pot voice that
encouraged all my choices: "Hey, girl, it's cool. I say go for it!"
That would be perfect if I was deciding whether to buy Girl
Guide Cookies but bad if I was wondering whether it's ok to
wear overalls after forty. And it turns plain dangerous when
I'm deciding what to say on stage.

ME: Hey, Kate Hudson, I'm not sure about going edgy tonight
at this church benefit.

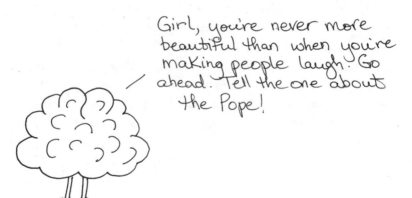

Girl, you're never more
beautiful than when you're
making people laugh. Go
ahead. Tell the one about
the Pope!

It was great to feel carefree finally. Risky, even. Especially because I had a show for international bankers coming
up. In the corporate world, high-end bankers are the most

terrifying audience. A lot of folded arms and smirks. The last time I had done an event like this I went into the audience to improvise with the guests and the first person I spoke to said loudly, "This is so stupid." The other audience members, well-groomed men in suits, stared at me stone-faced, as though signalling, "The group has spoken. Your act IS so stupid." A few days later my agent called to say the bankers loved the show and wanted to hire me back the next year. Apparently withholding approval is a good time in certain circles. Still, please put the word out that comedy is generally more enjoyable with arms uncrossed.

PAT: Will do.
ME: You're the best!

So, with filter disengaged, I arrived at the venue, where the bankers sat predictably with their arms crossed to defend against humour, and Kate-Hudson-on-pot started up again.

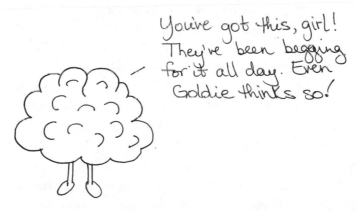

You've got this, girl! They've been begging for it all day. Even Goldie thinks so!

I took to the stage, smiling ear to ear like an idiot, for what I'd been told was a roast. Well, the event planner had asked for a roast, but the bank exec who hired the event planner wasn't aware of that instruction and had merely wanted a customized show with some jokes about banking. Five minutes into my act, I was on fire, berating every one of his guests while he stared, mouth agape.

"Lady, you picked the wrong day to wear a see-through top. Best way to break through the glass ceiling is to break into some appropriate clothing—am I right, fellas?!"

"Hey, buddy, anyone ever fall for those highlights? What colour is that—'midlife-crisis gold'?"

"What kind of last name is Furshuck—take away the middle part and what have you got? Go ahead, say the F-word with me, people!"

I should have known from back when my father was placed on that particular drug (within a month he dropped the F-word into a joke at church services) that it might not have been the best medication for a performer. I tried riffing with the bank head in the audience, but he just leaned close to my ear and spat out the words "When will you end this?!" Oblivious to the pained grimace on his sweaty red face (or my reputation as a clean comedian), I did a full hour and congratulated myself on my roasting prowess when I finished the show to modest applause. I was feeling so celebratory in fact that I gave Scott a bj in the green room 'cause Kate Hudson told me to! I felt less celebratory the next morning when my agent called to say that the executive described the show as the most humiliating experience of his career. I was flabbergasted and began defending myself, wondering why the pills picked this very moment to stop working.

ME: "Kate? Kate, where are you at, woman?!"

Gotta go.
— I have a thing.

When my agent asked what exactly I had said while improvising with the guests, a quick medley of all my worst moments from the night before flashed back to me. In the sober light of day, it was really embarrassing to repeat them, and I felt like I did when I was caught shoplifting from a drugstore in eighth grade and the officer made me tell what I had taken while my parents listened in. (Ironically, I was hired by that same chain for a show years later and felt a little sneaky cashing the cheque.)

The medication wasn't so awesome that it could handle shame: it just set you up to put your foot in your mouth but didn't mellow out the aftermath. I called my doctor the next morning and we made a plan to wean me off of it. A little anti-social behaviour seemed a small price to pay for avoiding more career-jeopardizing emasculations of bank heads. Back to being a socially paralyzed performer.

Where I need the invisibility cloak most is in smaller towns—towns with (ugh) manners. Most comedians have at least one other act on the bill when they're touring tiny towns; someone to commiserate with if your green room happens to be a hallway or if there's a buffet table on stage and people are nonchalantly helping themselves to food while you're telling jokes two feet away or if the audience is empty or maybe the audience is full but everyone is on their phone and completely ignoring you. You're relieved when you come off stage and there's a buddy there who can say, "I know the feeling!" But I'm almost always hired as a solo act. That's manageable when I'm healthy, but tricky when I'm depressed. And gut-wrenching when I'm depressed *and* anxious *and* flying to what I fear might be the world's chummiest hamlet.

ME: Read on, Pat. Read on if you dare!
PAT: Yup. That's ... that's what I'm doing.

I was invited to do a show in an area so isolated there's no road access during the summer (you can, however, reach it on ice roads in the winter. So Canadian, eh?). I flew to a nearby town and switched to an even tinier aircraft that I first assumed was a miniature cargo plane based on the folding seats and unsecured boxes jammed into the back rows. Everyone else aboard looked like they were just hopping casually on a subway to ride a few stops. One lady even had a homemade birthday cake on her lap, which I wished we could all have shared, given there was no cabin crew to hand out snacks (and despite all my hoping, the captain didn't put the plane on autopilot to hand out pretzels). Anyway, where introversion ends and pre-show reclusive ritual begins is sometimes a blurred line, but as we travelled farther north and each town appeared smaller than the last, a wave of social anxiety hit me and suddenly this pleasant destination seemed terrifyingly intimate.

There'll be nowhere to hide.

Their friendliness will suck the life force out of me.

I'll be nothing but a raisin by the time I get on stage!

In a failed effort to make myself less conspicuous, I twirled my obnoxiously yellow hair up under my H&M captain's hat (I had taken to wearing it after I put one on as a joke once and someone remarked, "It makes your head look smaller"), put on my gargantuan Olsen-twin-esque sunglasses, and tried to blend in.

I had requested through my agent that a taxi take me to the hotel, but the polite client insisted on doing the neighbourly thing and stood waiting for me at the mini-airport.

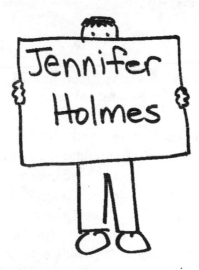

ME: Hi. Wow, thanks! I'm Jessica, actually, but no matter. Sorry for the inconvenience—I would gladly have taken a taxi.

CLIENT: There's no taxi service here.

ME: Oh, well, that's odd. Usually if a town's big enough for a hotel, it's big enough for taxis?

CLIENT: There's not a hotel.

ME: Oh, I was just given this address for my lodging. (*shows paper*) I guess it's more of a bed and breakfast?

CLIENT: There's no breakfast.

ME: So, it's someone's house, basically?

Yup, it was someone's house. A charming, single-storey pre-fab, as most homes up north are. When you're flying in from the nearest city, you start to notice you're no longer seeing square houses, but long rectangular bungalows with pastel aluminum siding. From up in the air, they look like Lego boxcars painted Easter colours.

See? Everything's fine.

I unpacked and showered, then headed for the sound check at the theatre, which turned out to be the community centre gymnasium. The sound check went off without a hitch 'cause it was just me putting my CD in their CD player. As I was wrapping up, the client informed me they had a lunch for me. I filled in the blanks in my mind to mean what I wanted it to mean—"There's a lunch waiting to be eaten by you"— instead of what it really was: "There's a lunch in your honour." I walked past the dozen or so people sitting around the buffet table in a clearing outside of the building, and nodded slightly at them without saying a word, then I wrapped a burger in a napkin and walked home. When I think of how ungrateful I must have appeared, especially after I visited the town grocery store and realized a head of lettuce costs upwards of $15, it makes me stare down at the floor with a tightening in my chest. I wish they could have known in that moment that it was nothing personal—I was just paralyzed with anxiety because Kate Hudson had stopped telling me what to do. With my stupid blond highlights, blazer, and heels (Who the hell wears heels to a sound check in a gymnasium anyway? I might as well have been Lady Gaga wearing a large Fabergé egg), I bet I looked like a snob thumbing her nose at them. It's not that I didn't want to be there: I wanted to be there and not be afraid.

Feeling a rush of pre-show adrenalin, my anxiety faded, and I walked back to the gym that evening with a little pep in my step. Only five people showed up for the show; maybe word had gotten out about my lunch snub. But the five who came were friendly people whose arms were uncrossed.

PAT: Congrats!
ME: Thanks!

On stage with the portable CD player, out of muscle memory I yelled, "Hit it!" then pushed the Play button myself. Twenty minutes into my set, my self-esteem took a dip when some kids walked in with a basketball and proceeded to start dribbling twenty feet from the stage. Unsure what the protocol was for mid-comedy sport interruptions, I put the mic down and asked one fifth of the audience, "Should I keep going?" and she replied, "Oh, for sure, they're just here to play ball," as though I wasn't sure what sport they were engaging in. More kids were arriving by the minute, and they were grabbing basketballs out of a storage closet. At no point did they organize themselves into teams, so it wasn't as though there was a game scheduled and my show happened to be interrupting it. They were just there to casually hang out despite the painted lady on stage trying to be heard over the *thud thud thud* of rubber on wood. Wanting to look like I was in on the joke, I tried to work it into my act and have my Russian character reason with them: "Hey, you boys, get over here and quit roughhousing. Don't make me sic the KGB on you." They ignored me, so I turned back to my quintet audience and sheepishly continued on with my jokes, wishing I was the one playing basketball while some other overdressed woman apologetically belted out show tunes. My adrenalin from being on stage has always lasted an hour or two after the show—this magical time when I feel grateful for my job, and grateful the anxiety has passed. I'll almost always go mingle with the audience for a drink when I come off stage. But that night I was exhausted from the day's worrying so I just thanked each of the five audience members and walked home.

On our drive back to the airport the next morning, feeling more human-like than on my arrival, I noticed the landscape for the first time: big raw boulders and miles of evergreens surrounding a pristine lake. "I should have gone for a hike," I thought to myself.

ME: It's incredibly beautiful up here. I really appreciated your committee choosing me. Big ol' thanks from this gal! Sorry that I couldn't draw more of a crowd.

CLIENT: We needed a laugh and we got one.

F#$k.

See, Pat? I really should get around to making that introvert T-shirt!

The Kids Are the Boss of Me

· · · · ·

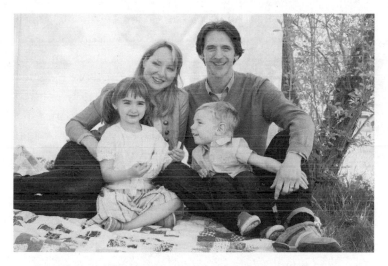

Credit: Kimberly Dunbar Photography

DON'T WE LOOK ok? This picture was taken during the beautiful time between my postpartum depression and second depression. I was in love with Scott, I felt close to the kids, and it was all a happy, if chaotic, adventure. But now imagine warped carnival music playing and the photo heating up and starting to melt as cheesy foreshadowing of what is to come, 'cause this is where it gets rocky. This is where I became less of a June Cleaver and more of a David-Hasselhoff-when-his-daughter-videotaped-him-lying-face-down-on-the-bathroom-floor-un-successfully-trying-to-eat-a-hamburger. Not my finest hour.

I can tell you that my kids actually had a blast for most of it, if you don't count a bunch of stuff. They were about three and four when I started to derail. They were my top priority and though I tried to shield them from my layabout ways, I had trouble hiding my angst. It started with guilt over being an absent mom. Not absent in the physical sense (I still signed up for many of the parent/child classes du jour—Mommy & Me Body Sculpting, Engineering for Tots, Baby Toastmasters, etc.) but just not being "present" during conversations. Remember when you were young, asking your dad one of those kid questions like "How come clouds are grey when water is clear?" and he replied "urmph" 'cause he was reading the paper and not really listening? "Urmph" was the only answer I could come up with, but I wasn't reading a paper, I was staring at the wall with an endless sea of worries:

Why are these kids always so chatty? Isn't the Baby Einstein
DVD providing them enough companionship?

Am I dressing age-appropriately? Why'd they make
"jumpsuits" in women's sizes if they don't want me
wearing them? I feel like an idiot!

I will never be finished doing laundry. I will die
under a pile of odd socks!

"Where's the friggin' finish line, Scott?" I'd ask, over-whelmed, even though I was just sitting there, shoulders scrunched up around my ears, white-knuckling my coffee cup. The kids asked questions in long, unpunctuated monologues. I'd still be processing "Hey, Mom, can we... " by the time they finished the sentence with "build a skating rink in the backyard?/Paint our shoes?/Live in the attic?" And though my response to most of these requests should have been "No, our yard is barely big enough to stand in/No, you painted your socks last week and now there's blue footprints all over the hardwood/No, it's nothing but fibreglass and squirrels up there," it's like my thoughts were made of soggy oatmeal and wouldn't fit into definitive answers. "Urmph" was the best I could do.

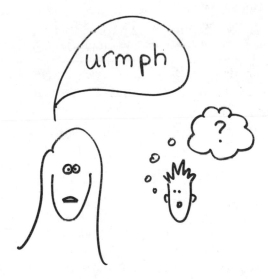

"Urmph" tided us over until Scott came home and gave the kids an answer in the form of words that actually appear in a dictionary. Indecisiveness is a symptom of depression. So is a lack of limit setting. If you can't set limits ("I love you so much I can't bear the thought of disappointing you") AND you're indecisive ("I haven't got any idea what to make for lunch—best if I make nothing, and have a hunger tantrum in two hours"), decisions are completely overwhelming. I've spoken with other moms battling depression who've also hit decision-walls in their own ways:

- staring at the laundry for three hours, unable to get started
- procrastinating from life by online shopping into a sea of debt, with most of the packages remaining unopened
- avoiding their kids because that's better than blowing up at them
- spending the whole day, every day, in bed, because they don't know what to do first
- surrounding the sofa with junk food so that it looks like a tornado hit a bodega (that one's me)

As my children's enthusiastic queries built up, I crumbled under the weight and said they had to limit their questions to three per day because I couldn't spare the hours it took me to debate the pros and cons of each request. Like I said, not my finest hour.

PAT: I'm not judging.
ME: Really? It gets worse.
PAT: Still not judging.
ME: You, Pat, are a rose among thorns. Thank you kindly!

I got most of my self-loathing and loafing out of the way during my Monday-to-Friday eight-hour lunch break that lasted from 9 to 5, when the kids were with the nanny or at school. Yes, by now there were four full-time scenarios for the kids:

1. Scott
2. Me, the stay-at-home mom who wasn't up to mothering

3. preschool and kindergarten
4. a full-time nanny

We hired our first nanny, a real go-getter, when Alexa was a few months old because I was working on a TV series with long hours. When I left the show beause I'd lost all enthusiasm for it, I still kept her on even though I only worked sporadically. Eventually she quit to find a job that entailed actual work and not just trying to stay out of the way in a house where the matriarch was like a grumpy bear going in and out of hibernation. I panicked.

What if the kids have to stay home from school
'cause of a cold or a school break?

I can't pretend to be ok for days at a time!

What will become of me?!

ME: We need to hire a full-time replacement now—it's an emergency!

SCOTT: Whoa. Even if we did need help, wouldn't it only be once in a blue moon?

ME: Oh, great. Now I have to look up whatever blue moons are! See? I have too much on my plate!

SCOTT: But it's a lot of money. Aren't there some great caregivers we can hire on an as-needed basis?

ME: We as-need someone full-time right now, just to be safe.

SCOTT: To be safe from what?

ME: Sorry, Scott, you've used up all your questions for the day.

We put out an ad on Kijiji for someone who didn't mind being a third wheel. Though there were plenty of great referrals for caregivers in our neighbourhood, I didn't want anyone local who might spill the beans about my sofa-tastic lifestyle. The first three nannies we interviewed had busy energies. One woman even tidied our living room throughout the interview, despite my half-hearted protest. Vivian* was the last of four applicants. She was warm and relaxed, and calmly explained she had moved to Canada to support her children, who remained with her mother in the Philippines. She wore jeans and sneakers and chewed gum casually throughout the interview. "Holy cow," I thought. "If she's treating this meeting like a movie theatre waiting line, surely she won't mind the irony of a mostly child-free nannying position!" We hired her immediately and she was just as chill as I'd hoped, never batting an eyelash over me sheepishly disappearing to idle in the basement every morning. Monday to Friday, she cooked and folded laundry and brought the kids on playdates when they were finished school and/or daycare. I was in awe of her. I myself had stopped arranging playdates. (I felt embarrassed by my constant late arrival; winded-ly rushing in only to turn back around because I'd forgotten the kids' water or hats or the kids themselves.) Meh, I was more comfortable alone anyway.

On weekends the kids quickly became the boss of me in our lawless house. Friday afternoon I'd start to get a little panicky.

ME: Why's there no school on weekends? I mean, what kind of a spoiled generation are we raising in this country when in some parts of the world, they're on a six-day school schedule so that moms can have more time to lie down and worry?

EMPTY ROOM: (*no answer*)

---

* Name changed.

Confrontation was my kryptonite, and soon enough my clever kids became more persistent. One weekend the dam that contained my guilt burst, and I abandoned urmphs for yeses. For every morning I slept through, every time I yelled, I tried to assuage my guilt and prove my love by giving in to their requests (even though it never actually decreased my guilt, so I can't necessarily brag that I'm a fast learner). Even though they were joyful, playful kids, I thought they needed persistent pick-me-ups to make up for having a part-time zombie for a mom. My logic was limited to asking myself, "Can this cause long-term damage?" And if the answer to that question was no, then my answer to the kids became yes!

"Mom, can I pee off the back porch?" Yes.

"Mom, can I bring a jar of pickles as my school lunch?" Yes.

"Mom, can I stay home from school this week?" Yes.

"Mom, can you kiss my wart better?" Gross! And yes.

My anxiety was the only thing that could evoke a "no." I had had, since their births, a full helicopter-parent worry system that made me fear open water, cars, long staircases, and men with moustaches. Those situations called for a definitive No! Well, a no, followed by yeses of placation.

"No. You're too young to walk by yourself to the park. But, here, take this tub of ice cream *and* my watch: both yours to keep!"

You might think, based on my ridiculous parenting style, that I had been raised in some back alley by a feral cat. But I actually have two amazing human parents! My mother and father are opposites in most ways, so I was raised in a dichotomous household.

PAT: Great word!

ME: Thanks. I googled it.

My dad, Randy, a Mormon computer fixer, encouraged risk taking—"instructions are for squares!"—while my mom, Laura, an agnostic feminist, did her best to ensure we reached adulthood safely "and with equal pay for equal work." My mother ignited my passion for learning; sitting with me for an hour while we listened to *Peter and the Wolf* on the record player, taking me to the library to look for books with strong female protagonists, and budgeting so I could go to a prestigious ballet camp every summer. My dad felt that our home was our camp, and why couldn't we turn the dining room into a greenhouse to grow our own indoor vegetable garden? He's got a rustic-mountain-man belief that we're all born with the answers and every one of us, including babies, just needs to face obstacles head-on in order for our survival instincts to kick in. Not only does he not sweat the small stuff, but like many members of our parents' generation, he kind of mocks anyone who does: "Haha ok, don't let the kids eat pencils, SURE."

The upside to his—hmmm, what's the opposite of heli-copter parenting?—parenting by natural selection was that he could turn mundane tasks into adventures. He took us shopping for groceries when my twin brothers, Marcus and George, were nine and I was seven. He had a long grocery list from my mom. He tore it in four, and handed us each a quarter of it. "Each of you get a cart. Get these items. Meet me back here in ten minutes." I have a rush now just thinking about it. I grabbed a cart, careful not to get one with the screwy wheel that steers you in the wrong direction, and set about hunting the dozen items on my list. Shoppers smiled inquisitively at this bony kid, all elbows and knees, with the giant cart, whiz-zing up and down the aisles. I said a quick sorry to everyone

I bumped into, the little Laura over my right shoulder whispering, "Don't talk to strangers." We unloaded our carts at checkout, exhilarated. Everyone had completed their list, with the exception of George, who had gotten Boo Berry cereal in place of Shredded Wheat, on purpose. My father wasn't mad. I was giddy on the drive home, my dad speeding up at every hill "so you feel it in your belly," and when we arrived home, we all excitedly told Mom about the grocery store challenge. She nodded. "Your dad is a fun guy."

He really is a fun guy! I just wouldn't ask him to babysit. It wasn't just 'cause he had my kids building a pyramid with 500 ml tins of canned food when they were toddlers. It was the game that followed that one, the game of Duct Tape Prisoners. The kids were delighted to be given the title of Escaped Convicts. Maybe that was a title with special sentimental value to my dad, given that almost forty years earlier, in that same backyard, he was being arrested for gun possession just after he'd been introduced to his future in-laws for the first time. "Oh ho ho, that Randy" is probably not what my grandparents thought while their eldest daughter's future husband was being forced into the police car, although when my dad tells the story he sure seems to think it was a laugh factory. The police realized the gun belonged to someone else and dropped the charges, but it was too late for a good first impression.

So right, Duct Tape Prisoners was underway, and both Alexa and Jordan laughed and laughed as they ran around trying not to get caught by Warden Randy, only bumping into a few table corners in their follies. It wasn't until the tape had to be removed that Randy said, "Uh oh." My ears perked right up and I paused my game on the iPad.

ME: Uh oh?

RANDY: Shoot, this tape really is as sticky as they say on the package!

To the kids' credit, they were very brave while we pulled the tape off. "This will make them tough in the long run," said the little Randy over my left shoulder.

So then playing was also off limits, unless a responsible adult was supervising Randy playing. There was still the odd moment when you'd think, "The kids are all in life jackets on the beach, and Randy's organizing a treasure hunt—what could go wrong? Surely I don't need to be right there the whole time." But then Randy buries the final treasure: a small hatchet. And only when four kids are digging happily in the sand, and one of them pulls out the treasure, triumphantly pumping it up in the air, yelling, "I found it! I found the weapon!" as the other kids dodge the swings, do you think, "Ok, I'll pay more attention."

My point is, whatever decision I made, I could picture half of my parents supporting it. There's a little Randy cheering "They'll have so much fun" over my left shoulder, and a little Laura pleading "Keep them safe" over my right. They both made such compelling arguments that I couldn't decide between the two.

The best decision is no decision!

My behaviour became predictable: placate, avoid, placate, avoid, power-bond, avoid, placate, blow up. My weekly grand finale was bawling on the sofa garbling, "I'm so sorry. No one did anything wrong. I'm just really stressed out."

Depression keeps parents from connecting with their children, regardless of how much they love them. What I wanted more than anything was for my choppy behaviour to cease and to instead reflect the steady and unconditional love I felt for my kids, but I kept spinning out of control. Alexa made this lovely "Scream Chart" to monitor who lost their sh#t the most, hoping it would encourage me to stay on the up and up.

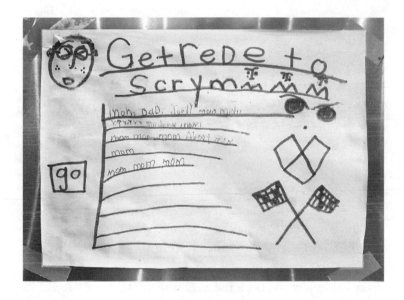

I was 75 percent embarrassed when I saw it, and 25 percent relieved that they had found a way to turn my outbursts into a kind of contest. In fact, if I could interview them back then about what their experience was like, I assume, in their resilience, they'd find a way to make it seem less bonkers than it actually was.

Bad Stuff	Good Stuff
• When she puts the trash can in front of her door, it means she had a "rough night" and we can't go in 'cause she's sleeping today.	• We have so many toys! Like, a mountain of them! Sometimes Mom looks at the mountain and shakes her head and says, "I'm a hoarder," so being a hoarder must be a super thing!
• Sometimes when we ask Mom a question, she has to look for the answer in a game of Jewel Mania on the iPad.	• Some families have green plants in their house. But we have brown, dry plants in every room. We're special!
• She'll wear an outfit one day, then wear it as pyjamas, and then stay in it the whole next day. But we're not allowed to do that.	• We don't have to clean up anything. Yesterday the cat barfed and Mom just put a cushion on it and went back to playing on the iPad.
• We told her how pretty she is and she just started crying, and then went to her room for a few hours.	• The TV is our second mom ☺

But those lists aren't a complete picture, because the kids don't remember the early ramifications. When I was in the thick of the depression and blaming all of my pain on Scott in a way I thought was secretive and undetectable, my son, Jordan, picked up on the resentment, and though he's sweet and cuddly and looks like a little yellow duckling, he would roll his eyes at Scott and ask "Why's he coming with us?" and "Why does he keep dropping things?"

The guiltier I felt for not being able to give them the best of me, the more I tried to make up for it by making every day like a trip to Disneyland, and the enabling culminated in me letting Alexa have eight friends sleep over for her sixth birthday party.

This will make everything better!

It was like trying to keep kittens in an open box. The movie and cake and manicures went ok, but it all went south at bedtime. All night they popped out of the rec room, one after another, waking me to report "so-and-so's nose is making a whistling sound," "I can smell the cat litter," "my pyjamas are pink," with the coup d'état being one poor little girl throwing up on the carpet at 5 a.m. After the final kid was picked up at 9:33 a.m. (those extra 180 seconds were excruciating!), my muscles were clenched as though I'd just escaped a tiger attack. I got on the sofa and didn't get up (except for bathroom breaks) for three days.

ME: Phew. That story winds me up every time! Don't worry. That was the peak. It's all resolution from here till the end of the chapter. You should get popcorn or something to celebrate making it over the hump.

PAT: Thanks. I'm good. I think it was worse for you than it was for me. 'Cause... I wasn't there.

ME: Right. Great! Where was I? Ah yes, depression!

Once I was diagnosed with depression I had to get hold of the reins again and figure out how to get the horses back in the stable. It took three sessions with Dr. Huh to accept that saying no to your kids isn't just ok, it's doing them a service.

ME: You're telling me that I should have said no when my six-year-old asked to have eight friends sleep over?

DR. HUH: Yes.

ME: And when my five-year-old asks to make naked snow angels in the backyard in the dead of winter?

DR. HUH: Yes.

ME: Won't the word "no" traumatize them? Shouldn't I at least offer a huge consolation prize so I can let them down easy? Like "No, you can't have a TV in your room, but here's three chocolate bars."

DR. HUH: No. They don't want a consolation prize. They want what they asked for. But you can still say no. "No" will give them boundaries, and that's what makes kids feel secure.

ME: You're basically telling me to be an a#*hole.

DR. HUH: (*sighing patiently*) If you say yes to everything, your children won't learn to self-soothe when faced with disappointment. They'll go out into the world as spoiled adults getting hurt every time they don't get their way.

ME: Oh. Well, how often can I say no?

DR. HUH: As often as no is the right answer.

ME: This all sounds like poppycock. I'll need to think about it. You're coming out of left field here with your crazy theories.

DR. HUH: Jess, I think we should increase the frequency of your visits.

I did start saying no. At first, I cringed when I said it, nervous that I was lobbing the emotional equivalent of a bowling ball at their fragile egos.

"No, you can't sleep in the car overnight." (*I'm such a jerk!*)

"No, you can't pour syrup in the bathtub." (*I'm gonna puke! That was so hard!*)

"No, you may not glue fun fur to my face." (*Why wouldn't Dr. Huh want me to give them $5 right now?? It would solve so much!*)

At first, they sulked and said I was mean. But after a few weeks of me disappointing them, they hadn't run away or exploded or whatever it was I was scared they'd do. They got used to hearing no, and within a few months, I could say it without dry heaving or avoiding eye contact. They stopped making constant outlandish requests. And as Dr. Huh predicted, they were more satisfied and secure than before. As a result, I was no longer crippled with fear of disappointing them. Well, riddled with fear, yes, but crippled with fear, not so much. Then, in a victory lap, I added chores (which is more trouble than it's worth because they scuff the walls with brooms and break dishes, but that's basically a rite of passage in childhood).

In addition to prescribing me a backbone, Dr. Huh suggested I get a dog so that I am forced to interrupt my 9-to-5 TV watching/crying schedule at least a few times every day. We got Ellie, a six-month-old mutt from a family that couldn't handle the needs of a puppy. She made me nervous, following me from room to room and staring at me for hours at a time while I lay on the sofa. When the kids came home, I'd pawn the dog off on them. "Can you please play with her? She's making me feel bad!" But I did get off the sofa for forty-five minutes every morning to walk her down a nearby trail. Turns out she wasn't so bad...

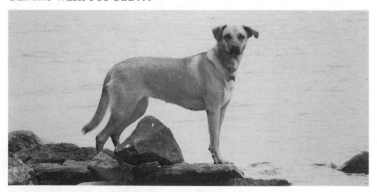

Ok, she's a total cutie-pants!

I was on new antidepressants that had me feeling slightly apathetic, and it was Randy who jumped back in the parenting seat and ordered the kids to ignore my directive that they could hook the wilfully disobedient puppy up to their scooters with rope to create a rolling sleigh. "Kids, untie that dog. Someone's gonna get hit by a car! You can tie each other up instead." Way to go, Randy! My point is, it takes a village. And sometimes in that village, the leaders take turns raising each other.

My mom (still the responsible one) sent me an article about how it's best for kids' mental health to get them to do the things that bring them happiness rather than to tell them to "feel" happy. It was good advice for adults, too. I loved Vivian, but she was like a get-out-of-jail-free card and I needed responsibility to motivate me to take care of myself (plus it turns out the bank hadn't been kidding about our debt), so we gave her notice and she was scooped up by a great family down the street.

Although my kids know I've been depressed, and I've explained it to them in layman's terms that eight- and ten-year-olds can grapple with, I'm waiting till they're older to elaborate. Maybe that's my next book:

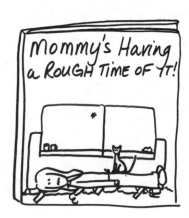

I still felt the need to make up for lost time, and dealt with that by following the kids around proclaiming, "See, Mommy loves being with you! Look at how close we are now!" which was awkward for all parties involved. Dr. Huh suggested mindfulness as a way to be in the moment with them, benefiting me both as a mother and as one of the tensest humans she'd ever met. I'm not sure I'm understanding mindfulness correctly because it seems too simple to be the cause of so much hoopla among the touchy-feely crowd, but as far as I can figure, you just pay attention to what's happening in and around you in the present moment without judging your reaction to it.

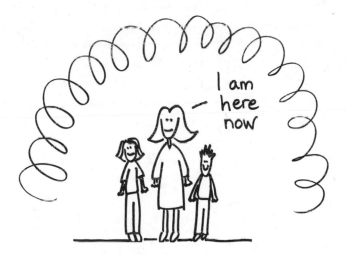

Although it interrupts my full-time hobby of worrying about the past and future, it does feel like there's this gift of connection just waiting for me anytime, anywhere. Even if I'm hurriedly applying sunscreen on the kids, wiping down the microwave from yet another burrito they've exploded, or fumbling with my camera and map instead of actually enjoying our weekend getaway in the country, I'll take notice of my breathing, of the expression on the kids' faces, of how soft their hands feel in mine, of the sound our shoes make on the ground. And suddenly I'm present, and not stuck in a loop between coming from someplace and going to another. If an anxious thought creeps in, I'll acknowledge it, and go back to my breathing and noticing and appreciating. And then when I step back on the roller coaster, I know I've got that moment tucked away to keep forever. On the superficial side, it lowers my hunched shoulders by about three inches (Tyra would approve!). Actually, mindfulness is useful to me everywhere except for at the dentist, where I feel it's important to visualize yourself as being anywhere but in the present.

The odd time I see scars left by those dark years; I sense my kids are scared of upsetting me, their armour going up even though I haven't yelled in years. I'll feel a twist of shame, then I'll remember my grampa's reassurance after my first game of adult soccer when I ran over and picked the ball up with my hands while my teammates glared at the mistake—"we do the best we can with what we know at the time"—and I'll acknowledge that I'm not a monster, but a person who was suffering and is earnestly striving to do better. My day is filled with gratitude for the simple joys of motherhood: Alexa pronouncing "potluck" "putt-lock" without realizing the error and Jordan explaining how he hopes he never gets better looking than he is now "'cause then even more girls will be after me!" I'm relieved to see the strong, compassionate people the kids are, perhaps despite it all. People often remark about how much Alexa looks like me. She has my features but with a Mediterranean flare. I asked my dad, "Does she remind you of me when I was that age?" And my dad said, "Just like you were at that age, but stronger," and a flood of relief poured over me.

What Comes First:
The Comedian or the
Depression?

. . . . .

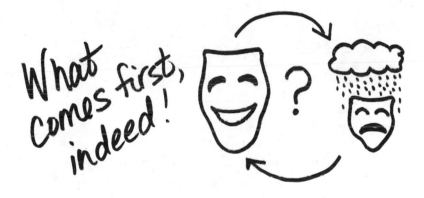

THE CHICKEN-AND-EGG DYNAMIC of depression and comedy is a real head-scratcher, and it's made me question whether comedy is the right place for me. I mean, are we screwy, unbalanced people drawn to this fly-by-the-seat-of-your-pants way of life, or does the feast-or-famine nature of the artist's way cause a few screws to come loose over the years? Researching this seems like a real long pain in the ass, so for brevity's sake I decided to instead ask a pro who's worked comedy clubs across North America. I sat down with Mike MacDonald (star of countless comedy specials and the movie *Mr. Nice Guy*) to see if he'd write this chapter for me—I MEAN, give me some insights.

ME: Thanks for doing this. You were at the top of my list.

MIKE: I'd hate to see the bottom. (*See? What a pro!*)

ME: So, I've noticed a fair number of comedians have suffered from depression at s—

MIKE: There are two types of comedians: diagnosed and undiagnosed.

ME: Yes! Is it because comedy's a double-edged sword—the thrill of making a crowd laugh versus the pain of going through a dry spell? Does depression make people funnier 'cause they've suffered or does comedy attract people that are predisposed?

MIKE: A bit of both.

ME: What makes us so loopy??

MIKE: Well, it's not a fair industry. I learned that the hard way. I'd taped my third stand-up special, and Letterman wouldn't have me on the show to promote it, even though I'd earned it. If you're the best at what you do, it doesn't matter. In sports, if you have a good player with good stats, he'll get on a team. But showbiz isn't like that. There's no talent + effort = certain advancement.

ME: Amen!

MIKE: It's subjective, and it's up to certain individuals who may or may not give you anything. The only consistency is that there is no consistency. And that's the hardest thing for someone with mental health issues.

ME: So you're confirming that comedy causes depression?

MIKE: I have so many RBIs comedically speaking. Ninety-nine percent of the shows I do, I get an *amazing* response, but I'm still not recognized for it. So I'll get pissed off.

ME: Right. Comedy isn't fair. One could even say it causes depression, right?

MIKE: My sitcom never got picked up even though it was considered a potential hit and starred a young Leo DiCaprio; my manager died three days after telling me he was gonna make me the next Steve Martin/John Candy (both of whom he had managed into stardom); and George Takei is credited for one of my jokes!

ME: Uh, what?

MIKE: Yeah. "Straight guys worry gay guys will treat them like *they* treat women." That's *my* line!

ME: Ouch. George owes you a fruit basket!

MIKE: An athlete can have an off day and it's a "bad game," but a comedian has a bad show and forever they'll think "they're not funny anymore."

ME: Yeah, I knew it was comedy's fault! Thanks a l—

ME: But then a joke'll pop in my head and all of a sudden the mood lifts. It's tough, but it's also my saving grace.

ME: Oh. (*pause, frown*) So you never thought of leaving comedy?

MIKE: To be what, a security guard? Nah, grass is always greener on the other side of the fence. When I find something funny, all is forgiven.

ME: So, basically, we're right back where we started.

MIKE: Well, I'm not gonna write your book for you.

Since Mike wouldn't write the book and we don't have all year, let's get some generalizations going: depression is caused by factors that are any combination of

a. biological (your neurotransmitters are sketchy and you'd best get to the pharmacy),
b. psychological (as a child you didn't learn to cope with negatives in a resilient way and you'd best figure out some coping mechanisms), and
c. environmental (you're experiencing job loss, social isolation, relationship conflict, chronic illness, or stressful working conditions, and you'd best find support and make some lifestyle changes).

I think comedians suffering from depression likely have a combo of the second and third, and if they're on the Deluxe Plan, a bit of the first one as well. We love deconstructing negatives: making jokes out of all the crap things that happen. It's like the garbage person—sorry, sanitation engineer: in order for you to live in a clean house, someone's gotta do the job of taking the diapers and apple cores off your curb and dropping them off in Michigan. We're your emotional garbage people!

Performing, writing jokes, that's the fun, rewarding part. The hard part is the downtime. You know the part of you that wakes up at 2 a.m. with irrational worries? That's the bulk of us comedians on a slow month. We're internalizers, thinking a mile a minute figuring out the equation of

What Really Happened + My Take On It = Joke

When life happens, we immediately want to frame it, give it context, ask "what does it mean" like we're a lonely teenager and our career is the captain of the football team who just texted us "s'up?" That's terrific if you're on stage looking for laughs, but destructive if you're sitting home watching one job after another go to your peers. Even outside of my depression, every time I had a career slump it would send me into an existential despair. Last month, Genna and I were sitting down together pondering what we're meant to do next, creatively speaking, and discussing whether a dry spell meant failed potential or was that just our inner muse giving us downtime to soak up more inspiration from life experience? Her husband, Anson, piped up: "See, I just always approached career from the viewpoint of 'Who can I get to hire me?' and went from there." We stared at him till he awkwardly left the table and picked up a guitar in the corner. That is not how we're built, despite the fact that I have certain jealousy over my brother, who drives a bus and comes home at the end of a shift NOT asking himself, "Did I have what they were looking for? What could I have done better? Do the other drivers respect my work?"

Environmental is the biggie. Rejection is a daily occurrence, and TV roles for women over forty dry up faster than a California raisin in a mid-August drought (sorry, that's the *Dr. Phil* viewer in me talking). I am one of the most requested speakers in my field, and—

PAT: In your field in Canada.
ME: Yes, Pat, in my field in Canada.

—and I still see my fair share of tumbleweeds. A breakdown went out a few years ago for "a Jessica Holmes type." I asked my agent if I could audition for the role and after making a call, he said, "Sorry, Jess, they're not interested."

Rejection stings, even though I only began this career as a hobby. One night at a campus bar, after a few Long Island iced teas, between Spirit of the West songs, a few friends and I dared each other to try stand-up. I was passionate about comedy, as a spectator only, and found the first experience terrifying. On my way up to the stage, my legs buckled and I swiped a stranger's drink for courage. The bright lights blinded me and I felt like I'd been breathing helium balloons all day. I pulled the mic out of the stand too zestily and banged myself in the mouth with it. I could feel my top lip starting to warm up and swell. But then I got a few lines out and got my first laugh. And just like that, I was hooked. For the next two years I jubilantly hopped on stage at every open mic night I could find, dodging the odd beer bottle, and performing for crowds of two while blowing my temp work paycheques on Second City classes.

Starving artistry, here I come!

I had a reputation for being a bit of a teacher's pet: I didn't have a hard childhood, I wasn't skeptical or sarcastic, and I quoted Oprah often. When I bombed I'd retreat backstage, swoop my arms in a big circle, and chant Dr. John Gray's mantra "O glorious future, come unto me" while my peers watched, a disparaging "Who farted?" look on their faces. Some of them had tough childhoods or a skeptical view of life that they cathartically channelled into their routine. They might have felt that I hadn't come by comedy honestly, that I was an impostor. "I hate your enthusiasm" was something I heard on a regular basis, followed by "Who do you think you are?" Offering those jaded comics a copy of my favourite book, *The 7 Habits of Highly Effective People*, "so you can shine your light, too," simply contributed to my reputation of being obnoxiously saccharine. But I was still glowing from the pride of completing an eighteen-month mission in Venezuela for the Mormon Church, and the eye rolls were wasted on me.

I had given comedy a two-year window, telling myself that if I didn't book something (beyond the arty black-and-white student film that featured only my hands) within that time, I'd find a different career path where I would actually get to DO the job. I was auditioning for everything, learning my lines on public transit, leaving my admin job at the Canadian Broadcasting Centre during lunch hour for "another doctor's appointment," never minding that it was costing me more to get to and from the auditions than I'd seemingly ever make back. At the twenty-three-month mark, my agent emailed me with an audition for a series of two-minute vignettes on a kids' channel. Entertaining a few people behind a desk was way less intimidating than getting a bar full of jaded arm-crossers to bust a gut, so I felt relaxed going in.

PRODUCER: Hi. Show us what you've prepared.
ME: Uh, prepared… how?
PRODUCER: Didn't your agent give you our notes?
ME: Shoot. No. Um, just a time and a place. Should I do some host-y stuff? (*jazz hands*)
(*SILENCE*)
PRODUCER: Go out and take a look at this sheet. Come back in five minutes and show us what you've got. Or don't.
ME: Thank you so much. I'll be right back.

The instructions were to be an unspeaking two-year-old learning to do kid things: planting a seed, blowing up a balloon, riding a teeter-totter. I went back in the room and became an oversized toddler, complete with big eyes, grunts, and giant gestures.

PRODUCER: Thanks for your time.
ME: It was my pleasure. Really.

And I raced back to the CBC in time to tell my boss, "The doctor says I'm still fine." A few days later my agent called to say that they were hiring me to play Little Big Kid.

O.M.G.!!!!!!!!!!

I speed-walked over to my friend Coretta's desk and explained the amazing news.

ME: I'm gonna be a star!
CORETTA: Oh, did you get on *MADtv*?
ME: No, a Canadian kids' show!
CORETTA: Jess, you booked a series? That's wonderful.
ME: Well, not a series, actually. They're calling it interstitials:
    two-minute clips that will play during commercial breaks.
CORETTA: Congratulations on . . . what you just described!

The workers I did scheduling for at the CBC had just gone on strike, so my boss had no problem giving me the time off of pretending I had something to do at the office. My agent informed me I'd earn $3,000 for a month's work (basically, that I was rich) and that night I bought non-generic-brand meat for dinner to celebrate with Scott.

The shoot, though a small production by industry standards, was my first taste of catered lunches, the spa-like decadence of sitting in the makeup chair, and the bliss of making people laugh by being my screwball self on TV. I happy-cried just enough times to make people feel awkward around me. On our final day of shooting, the producers gave me a big bouquet of flowers, and my mouth hurt from smiling like a pageant queen. Friends joked about how embarrassing it must have been to play a clowny toddler, but I was thrilled. Over the next few years, I was lucky enough to perform and write on one series after another, loving every minute of creating new characters.

When I was giving it my all on TV, I felt special, and special is not a good feeling to chase. Special is fleeting. Special, like its cousin important, are both tough to duplicate and based largely on your value to other people. When special ends, as it did when my five-back-to-back-series spree ended, all of that deep thinking that helps a comedian come up with jokes on the fly became my worst enemy. I couldn't see the positives, only the rejection, no matter how much I chanted and swooped my arms like a g$#%$mn helicopter. On paper I still had a charmed life: I got hired on average once every few weeks to show up at a convention centre or hotel to sing and tell jokes for [insert bank/car company/retailer]'s AGM. It's very rewarding work, but... it's not really a job. I mean, I'd never even heard of "corporate comedian," have you?

PAT: No. (*pause*) Oh, wait, was that a hypothetical question?
ME: Yes, but I love your enthusiasm!

With every performance I'd think, "These gigs are too good to be true. I'm not as funny as the competition. I have nothing to fall back on when my luck runs out!" Some weeks I'd get hired almost every day, and then three months would go by with no paid work. My annual income is like a yoyo in the wind, which my accountant describes as "a delightful challenge." One year, Scott and I are buying a car and planning a holiday, and the next, we're putting out ads for basement tenants and selling old clothes on eBay (which I don't recommend unless you have the patience to answer thirty buyer questions before selling a $3 pair of cargo shorts).

I was reading *The Secret* when I started this journey. "Just visualize what you want, and it will appear." When I visualized, then became successful, it imprinted on me that it was my attitude that led to my success. And when I kept believing with all my might, but the TV roles ended, I blamed myself for not having enough faith, or enough "it factor." It kind of reminds me of the story my mom told me about how she and my uncle would torment their little brother Pete by unhooking the cable in the basement when Pete watched TV. He would get frustrated, and when they heard him bang on the box, they'd plug it back in. After doing this many days in a row, Pete believed that banging the box was responsible for fixing the TV. Years later, when the cable went out in his house, he would bang his TV and feel deflated that he had lost his power to fix things with sheer Fonzie-ness.

PAT: Is Pete bitter about it?
ME: Maybe, but out of that bitterness came his great sense of humour, so win-win!
PAT: That's actually lose-win.
ME: So it is!

Between my lack of creative purpose, chronic insomnia, and a handful of psychological factors, some part of me broke, and I went from being a healthy person who was down about her career to being a depressed person who was down about everything. My new hobby was watching other comedians be more successful than me on TV. TV—who I thought was my ally, my buddy—now took the peers who out-it-factored me and rubbed them in my face. I had to start watching American reality TV just to make sure I didn't see any familiar faces. I'd ruminate over the fact that I wasn't enough, looping back over my problems like a broken record.

I've wasted my career.

People are embarrassed for me.

Does everyone's belly-button lint smell terrible, or is it just mine? And why do I keep sniffing it?! I'm the worst!

It made me tired within minutes of waking up. On average, during my two years of depression, my day went like this:

9 a.m. Tired from another night of iffy sleep, start the day with TV.

10 a.m. Check email. See invitation to hang out, but think, "Wouldn't my time be better spent actually working on my career?" Decline invitation and *also* don't work on career.

11 a.m. Eat in front of TV.

12 p.m. Cry in front of TV.

1 p.m. Sleep in front of TV.

2 p.m. Make salad. Chase it down with half a box of cookies. Cry again.

3 p.m. Play Candy Crush.

4 p.m. Watch TV. Contemplate how our ancestors procrastinated. "Oh, that I hadn't idled away the day rolling hoops and making eyes at cousin Barnabas!" Feel tingle at finding kernel of joke. Panic at wasted day. Desperately beg agent to submit me for anything, including hand-only student films.

5 p.m. Kids home. Tell them I had a good day at work.

Some observations about this timeline:

- **Any NBD (Never Been Depressed) person would ask, "Well, why don't you just get out there and do something?"** One of the most prevalent symptoms of depression is not feeling like doing anything, ever. It's like asking a smoker, "Well, why don't you just chew gum instead?" We're not stupid, we're stuck—in my case under an imaginary Looney Tunes–style anvil.

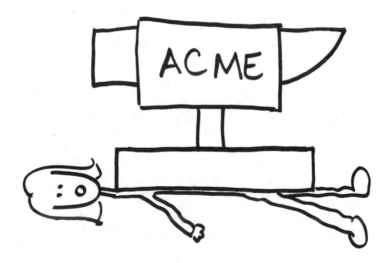

- **I *was* trying.** At times I did use every ounce of willpower I had to start my own projects, even creating a series of healthy web videos one month. I was exercising, showering daily (very big deal!), doing my hair, and having Scott tape the segments with three seconds' notice ("I don't care if you're on the toilet! Pinch it off and record me before my coffee high is over!"). The videos peaked at about fifty views each. The disappointment of being less popular than a talking orange reinforced my belief that I was untalented, and better off not trying.

- **Sometimes I jump the shark.** The term comes from a book about the season-five episode of *Happy Days* where The Fonz (yes, it's a two-Fonzie-reference chapter!) has to water-ski over a shark in order to [doesn't matter]. It means being desperate to stay in the game, something I can identify with when corporate work slows down every summer. Looking for work in August is like looking for your soulmate at 2 a.m. when the bartender yells, "Last call." You end up with a real loser, or in my case, a clowning routine at a stranger's birthday party. You know when you see some celebrity doing an adult diaper commercial and you think, "Wow, they must need the money"? It's more likely they got the request on a slow day when they were antsy about being out of the spotlight. "I still matter, right?" And, sure, they probably DO need the money to pay off a scorned assistant/buy another endangered pet leopard/ have their neck stapled to the back of their ears (or whatever that operation is that makes your face look like a shiny drum head).

- **I crumble under the pressure of an unscheduled day.** When there is no clear answer to "What's the best use of my time?" I panic about making the wrong choice, and decide it's safest to just curl into a ball and let the sound of *The Real Housewives* drown out my worries.

One of my first thoughts after being diagnosed with depression was, "This isn't the right job for me." I asked Dr. Huh if I should abandon this career altogether rather than try to fix every aspect of it, sort of like when I had lice and my father buzzed off all my hair 'cause that was less inconvenient than my mom having to take a day off work to pick nits.

DR. HUH: Do you feel it needs to be all or nothing?
ME: Well, the buzz cut worked. Lice-free for twenty years!
DR. HUH: Hair grows back.
ME: Touché, Dr. Huh!
DR. HUH: What did you call me?
ME: Nothing!

We explored whether it made more sense to stay in a volatile career that fulfills me (sometimes) versus looking for a new career where I'd still face obstacles but where I could hope to feel useful forty hours a week, or at least where one of the job requirements would be "not pitying oneself on a sofa all day." I had heard author Miriam Toews say, "I have stories to write, and if that means living in a tent in someone's backyard, so be it." I doubted I was as virtuous when it came to comedy. One daddy-long-legs in the tent and I'd start handing out resumés. I turned to Genna for wisdom.

ME: G, what the f#$k do I do?
GENNA: Well, what would you tell your kids if they wanted to go into comedy?
ME: That it's the career equivalent of playing scratch-and-win lottery tickets.
GENNA: C'mon, J.
ME: It's true! Do you remember Edie Falco winning that award that time?
GENNA: No.

ME: She said she was grateful for the win, but that it didn't carry much weight because she has so many talented friends who are just as hard-working who don't get series and who don't win awards. I'd encourage my kids to work someplace where if you work hard, you'll see a payoff. There are lots of ways to be creative in life without making it your job.

GENNA: Sure, but—

ME: Wait, I'm on a roll. I'd warn them, "Sometimes actors don't get the job because one eye is smaller than the other or their voice is too nasal or they aren't very good at networking or they don't have that elusive thing that keeps 3 percent of actors working and the rest waiting tables and temping and hoping. BUT... if it's really, really something someone feels they need to try, they should go for it. They should work hard and be polite and even a little ballsy, and maybe they'll make it." It could happen.

GENNA: It happened for you.

ME: (*pause*) I guess. Kinda. Then why isn't this any fun? Why is Robin Williams gone? Why is the suicide rate for artists twice as high as for the rest of the population?

GENNA: Listen, I just came over to ask if you wanted to go for a pedi and read *People Magazine*, so...

The ruminating that comedians do, the instability, the competition, it all adds up. Maybe the same way that it's a virus that causes colds, but you're more likely to be susceptible to that cold if you eat nothing but delicious bonbons and poutine and get no sleep, some jobs add to your susceptibility. But even if, way back when I was still in university, a doctor had diagnosed me as "too sensitive" and handed me a prescription to prevent depression that read, "Avoid comedy. Try something stable. And probably avoid magic and mime as well, just to be safe," I'd still have had the wanderlust to take on this challenge.

Still, I'm so unhappy. I love making people laugh, but not enough to suffer like this.

The right answer—for me, at least—wasn't to walk away… yet. I stood up, looked depression in the eye (ok, it was just me in my basement talking to the air while the cat cleaned herself at my feet), and proclaimed, "It'll take more than that to stop me, probably!"

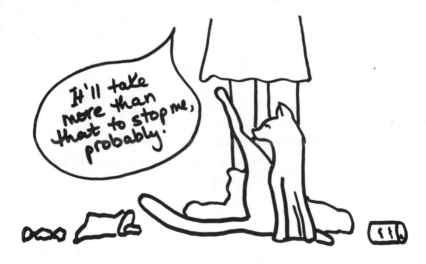

I took some time to explore ways I could make comedy a healthier place for me (above and beyond the therapy and medication, which seemed to be building upward momentum)—

tools that could stop me from ruminating when it gets hard, and make my career about goals that are independent of success (like reducing the stigma of mental health or getting people to eventually stop saying, "You know, for a woman, you're really funny"). Here's what's working for me so far:

1: Reminding myself it's nothing personal. I was emceeing a tech symposium in Montreal and Billy Baldwin was a guest speaker doing a Q & A about how being an actor relates to being an entrepreneur. He had taken a light interest in the business after his brother Alec found success and Billy booked the movie *Born on the Fourth of July* on his second audition. He starred in eight movies back to back. And then... his phone stopped ringing so much. He described show business as a double-edged sword that "sells an illusion that's barely attainable and almost never sustainable," and said that out of all the Screen Actors Guild members, 97 percent earn less than $20,000 per year for their acting. If there's a slow couple of months, maybe it's nothing personal. Maybe it's just math.

PAT: And Billy? What happened to Billy?!
ME: Well, he ended his speech by saying he's had to think outside of the box and reinvent himself in order to support his family, so now he's acting and producing and speaking. He was a barrel of laughs backstage. When he heard me mistakenly ask one of the producers of the show, "Are you with the band?" he joked, "Don't you hate when you get yourself kicked off next year's symposium?"

2: Realizing the grass is *not* always greener on the other side of the fence. My job might have pitfalls, but it's not like being a politician, or a farmer, or that person who empties other people's septic tanks is depression-proof. Even if I found the stability and usefulness I crave in another line of work, maybe there'd be longer hours, mandatory awkward team-building challenges, "that guy" in the next cubicle who's always microwaving fish and forwarding inappropriate emails. One of my neighbours left the competitive world of dance to become a teacher. One day when I was griping to her about work stress, she said, "Oh my God, I just assumed you had it all!" and I had been thinking the same thing about her. My side of the fence might have patchy grass, but it also yields a fresh crop of road trips and diva wigs each spring.

3: Not keeping up with the Joneses. Or the Heffernans. Or anyone. Racehorses have blinders put on so that they won't get psyched out when the competition pulls ahead. I needed my own little blinders to stop comparing myself to others. I started by curbing the time I spend on Facebook, which is like a faulty time-travel machine: you go online for five fun minutes, and suddenly it's an hour later and you feel like everyone's life looks better than yours. So now I treat social media like a hot tub: get in and get out before you catch something! And I'm trying to be less defensive when people ask, "What projects are you working on?" I was embarrassed to say "I'm waiting to be in demand" so I'd panic and say something like "I'm taking a break from acting while I work on projects closer to my heart like ... getting that 'off-leash cat park' going." But I'd rather be honest than important, so now I answer, "I'm working here and there, raising my kids, and trying to find the source of a lingering sulphur smell in our basement closet."

4: Creating stability. Since no two days are alike and my schedule is unstable, my psychiatrist recommended I start doing daily things that give my life structure, like playing team sports

(I was already playing basketball once a week, and I joined a soccer league where, so far, my go-to move is passing the ball to the opposing team) and getting that dog I mentioned one chapter ago. The dog was the best suggestion 'cause a) I'm her hero and b) when I realized what the dog walker cost, I took up jogging so I could exercise her for free. And I make myself write every day—could be mining new material for stand-up, researching positive psychology for a keynote, or composing a song that will only get fifty views but makes me laugh. Oh, and I get one hour of TV per day. Do you hear me, Jessica? One hour! (That one's a work in progress.) When I'm pushing myself, there's no inclination to stop and ask, "Am I enough?" In fact, the question seems so stupid now. If I'm going to stop and ask anything, it's "Where's the jerky at?"

5: Actually working. I'm a different person when I'm working. I can even feel my energy increase with every hour I'm productive. If I hadn't convinced myself I should be special or nothing, I would have realized there's a middle ground. The other day I turned down an offer from my agent because "it's not my dream job" and she replied, "Work begets work. Start working on this and before you know it, other offers will come in." And she's right. The same thing goes for relationships. And fitness. If you just get in the game, start putting some energy into that area of your life, a momentum starts building. My friend Jody Vance once gave me the advice "Do the thing to do the thing." It means if fatigue or procrastination or anxiety are keeping you from making a choice about what to do, just start doing something, anything, and then you've built up the momentum to do the thing that you actually wanted to do in the first place. Even getting off the sofa and doing ten minutes of work or exercise or plant-watering can save me from spending the next four hours watching daytime television, getting invested in the outcome of strangers' paternity tests and makeovers. I have to stop asking myself, "What does it all mean?" and just start moving. To borrow a line from Britney Spears: "Work, b^&ch."

6: Chasing helpful, not special. Eckhart Tolle says (and I'm really paraphrasing here) don't chase being special; chase being useful with whatever talents you have, and that's where fulfillment comes from. Thinking "I want to be of use in any way I can" is a much deeper, psychologically sustainable mindset than my early career philosophy of "I'm so lucky! I've got a gift!" In fact, backstage at that Billy Baldwin event, Chynna Phillips, his wife of twenty-seven years (188 in Hollywood years), was getting ready to sing her Wilson Phillips hit "Hold On" and I heard her praying, "Let me reach whoever needs it." I asked her about it (we had power-bonded when I flatironed her hair a minute earlier) and she said, "I need to attach singing to a higher purpose or I get all up in my head."

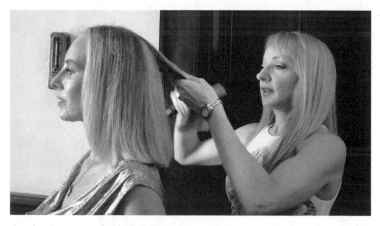

Credit: Courtesy of my phone.

I realized we have to use a lot of Jedi mind tricks to channel major chutzpa on stage while still staying humble enough to not sweat bouts of unemployment. And being attached to a higher purpose would help. Scott and I had been going to Unitarian church (like TED Talks for environmentally conscientious agnostics) on and off for a few years, and I try to attend once a month now, to get grounded and inspired. I finally acknowledged that being a "corporate comedian" is indeed a job, and committed that leg of my career to reducing the stigma of mental illness. I try to see each show as a chance to spread a positive message and push myself creatively, instead of "phew, more proof I'm still not unemployed!"

I tried those new approaches. I tried them again and again. And although no single one of them "fixed" me, in various combinations they make me more resilient and able to enjoy the ride. When I recovered from depression, the fog lifted, and I could see how fortunate I was to even have a job, let alone earn a living expressing myself. No, I'm not at the top, but I'm a close 1,002nd, and that's still a long way from where I began.

It feels so good to be grateful again.

There are, of course, still cringe-worthy moments. Last Canada Day, I was asked to emcee an event in Ottawa where a popular band would be the headliners. The event was spectacularly glamorous and I was whooping it up with the crowd. During a break, the band's manager came over and said, "The band would like you to join them on stage to sing the last song of the night together." I replied with a delighted "Yes!" 'cause singing ok-ish is something I do great!

Honestly, how blessed am I??

An hour later, when the band announced they were doing their final song, I hopped up on stage.

Silence.

Everyone on stage turned and looked at me. The lead singer whispered something to the guy beside him, who walked across the stage to me and whispered, "What's your name?"

I think I'm gonna throw up.

"Uh, Jessica," I whispered back, and he walked quietly back as the audience stared, and whispered to the lead singer, who finally announced, "And here's Jessica."

It was embarrassing, but I didn't shrink back onto the blue sofa. I cringed briefly, then shrugged it off, and sang along to the band's final song. A day later I was re-enacting it for my friends, all of us laughing. Mike was right. When you find the funny, all is forgiven.

*I don't blame you, comedy. I just think I got
to be a little too dependent on you.*

Last year, I picked a lane. I decided to say, "I choose comedy," instead of wondering daily whether I should bail on this industry and instead open that all-gluten bakery I've been dreaming of. Yes, it's a volatile industry with highs and lows that read like a day trader's EKG printout, and, yes, some of us are a li'l more susceptible than others, but I'm going all in anyway; let the chips fall where they may. Mmmm chips. Lord, am I snacky!...

PAT: Uh, Jess, were you going somewhere with that?
ME: No, that's it. That's the end of the chapter.
PAT: Ok. Just checking.

So Here's the Thing

· · · · ·

WHEN I WAS a kid, my mom brought me to watch the Ottawa marathon, even though we didn't know anyone running in it. I was used to her bringing me to smart places on weekends— libraries, art galleries, ballets—always armed with "mom snacks" like orange slices or raisins or cut-up pieces of cheese in Kleenex. She'd hold the snack out a few inches in front of me, and without looking I'd pull the bits of tissue off and pop the food in my mouth. We settled in a shady spot near the Bank Street Bridge and she pulled out some cucumber slices with tissue stuck to every surface.

ME: Why are people clapping?
MOM: Because the runners are working so hard. We're cheering them on.
ME: Even the slow runners?
MOM: Yup.

We watched for hours in what must have been a new record for me not asking "Can we go now?" I clapped as loudly as I could, even throwing in a few self-conscious "woo-hoos." We cheered for the fittest athletes leading the pack, then we cheered for the middlers, and then, after minutes went by with no runners, we cheered for the sparse trotters bringing up the rear. Some were half-walking, some were very old, or very scrawny, but they all kept moving. I wondered what had brought them to this place where they wanted to take on this task, even knowing they'd likely be the last ones to finish. I felt a lump in my throat when I thought about their tenacity. I leaned into my mom and cried.

BETWEEN MY POSTPARTUM depression and my second depression, at a time when I was feeling joyous and carefree, I was cast in a live musical. Musical theatre folk are enthusiastically chummy, I assume because singing and skipping and wearing rouge boosts serotonin. The cast was so friendly in fact that on our first break together, after people excitedly introduced themselves and peppered me with questions, I leaned over and asked one of the other performers, "Are they mocking me?" I became fast friends with one of the gentlemen working on the show—an irreverent type whose sardonic jabs would make amazing bumper stickers. He opened up to a few of us about the difficult time he was going through. He was getting counselling but his doctor had also prescribed him antidepressants. Though he was desperate to start taking them, he was also too discouraged to actually fill the prescription (very common in depression: knowing exactly what you should do, but feeling too stuck to make the leap). Lately he had barely wanted to get out of bed, let alone run errands. We each shared our mental health experiences with him (like I told ya, most artists have one), and he decided to get the prescription filled. The three of us followed him to the pharmacy, chanting his name and singing the *Rocky* theme song along the way. Waiting at the counter, we acted out anti-depressant commercials:

"I just grew a family!"

"Suddenly, I'm on a luxury vacation!"

"I never noticed the ocean before!"

At rehearsal the next day, he sarcastically announced, "I feel like myself again. The colours are so much brighter already!" The pills didn't work that fast, but they might have eventually made an excruciating period more bearable. Or maybe they had the placebo effect and just made him feel stronger? Whatever the case, today he's a seemingly content guy and he tells me about his new girlfriend and latest creative endeavour when I see him at yoga. It's as though that blip in his time line was just a passing anomaly, like a flu that came and went.

But not all depressions are equal.

While I believe medication helped greatly with my PPD, this time 'round, to borrow a medical term, it wasn't doing diddly-squat. Well, diddly-squat is an exaggeration; perhaps half-a-squat or diddly-some is more accurate, but pills alone weren't saving me from the sofa. And just like when Jude Law cheated on Sienna Miller and she was torn because "he broke my heart, but he's also my best mate," I was stuck lying on this $%#* sectional that filled me with self-loathing but was also my safety net. My lifestyle needed an overhaul. Above and beyond the changes I mentioned in the previous chapter, I made new efforts that regular folk might have called "cute" but that felt to me like I was bench-pressing a hundred. (For the record I don't know what people are referring to when they say they can bench-press a hundred. Is it pounds? Kilos? Garlic?) Nevertheless, I felt more like a boss with each tiny accomplishment. The hardest part was actually getting started, and I remembered my grandmother always counting to three before she got out of her seat.

ME: What happens if you don't count to three?
GRANDMOTHER: Well, I don't get up, of course!

That was logic enough for me and it became my habit: counting to three to make myself start some menial task that seemed as daunting as jumping off a dock into icy cold water.
"1-2-3" Get off the sofa.
"1-2-3" Make a phone call I've been procrastinating doing.
"1-2-3" Ignore the promotional emails that promise a quick fix and get to work on something.

PAT: Even when an email headline reads, "Final Hours! 30% off!"
ME: Even then, Pat. Even when it says, "Last Chance for Early Access!" Which I've realized means the same sh*t will still be on sale tomorrow. I don't take the bait!
PAT: Respect.
ME: . . . well I *usually* don't take the bait.
PAT: Still, I'd give you a participation badge for that!

Jogging (albeit a slow jaunt to the park and back in jeggings and floppy sun hat while the dog pulls as far away from me on the leash as she can) made me feel strong. Within a few months, I had broken the 1K mark, and was now jogging for longer than five minutes before giving up and ducking into the nearest dollar store for a candy bar and tabloid magazine. I finally invested in proper fitness gear (after a neighbour commented, "Not a ton of wicking on denim, huh?"). Also, I guess a lady running in jeans and a wool sweater while her dog jerks her left and right looks like she's in some kind of trouble, and good Samaritans were pulling over from time to time to offer me a lift wherever I was trying to get in such a hurry, so I upgraded to a convincing pair of lululemon knock-offs. Even the dog, perhaps seeing my new running gear as a sign of competence, began to run at pace beside me.

Feeling basically like an Olympic hopeful in the imaginary 3K event motivated me to abandon the "depression diet," which is all about the instant gratification of "sorta" food because you just want a fast fix versus actual food, even though it meant I'd no longer get to defensively exclaim, "What kind of loser eats squash??" at the grocery store.

Sorta Food	Actual Food
any item whose ingredients you can't pronounce	anything grown
meals whose directions include "Then you just put it in the microwave for ten minutes, Styrofoam container and all!"	things that take at least five minutes to prepare (you're worth the trouble, air-popped popcorn!)
packaging with limited foods (I'm talking to you, centre aisles!)	foods with limited packaging (nice to meet you, veggies!)

I even switched from regular coffee to decaf 'cause half-way into my first cup of the real stuff, after an enthusiastic poop, I'd zestfully proclaim, "I'm gonna write a one-woman show where I play *all* the characters in *Star Wars*!" then crash twenty minutes later. And of course there are still treats. On Halloween proper, my kids eat some loot, but at the end of the night they pour out their bags and pick their thirty favourite pieces to eat over the next thirty days. I tell them that the rest of the candy is going to "needy families" and then discreetly put it in the cupboard, way high up, so I can sneak it into the movies with me.

PAT: You sneak food into the movies?

ME: Only little treats 'cause I don't want to buy the eight-pound bag of sugar and food colouring they sell at the concession stand. And fine, I did sneak in actual food once. They were elk pepperettes and—

PAT: Elk? Like the guys that pull Santa's sled?

ME: Those are reindeer. These are their cousins. Anyway, we'd been at some organic food market and the guy at the elk meat booth said it was more ethical and lower fat than beef and he was so sure of himself when he proclaimed "that's the elk difference" that I bought a pack of elk pepperettes and stuck them in my bag and remembered them a few days later when we were at the movies. I didn't have scissors so I chewed open the package while Scott watched, turned off, and that's when an old, greasy, cured meat smell wafted up quickly and aggressively, exaggerated by the lack of refrigeration (which I didn't think dried meat required!), causing a few patrons in neighbouring seats to complain loudly. Even Scott moved three seats over, despite me explaining "that's the elk difference." So anyway, yes, a mini pack of Smarties seems like an ok thing to sneak into a theatre, right?

PAT: (*silence*)

ME: Right, Pat?

PAT: Sure. Of course.

My non-movie treat is pie. The joy of pinching the edges of the crust, and pouring in apples, peaches, or blueberries with cinnamon and a little maple syrup we buy right from the sugar shack—it's kind of a Zen moment for me and the closest

I may ever get to meditating. For the record, I tried meditation at least three times for about two minutes each, then I just got frustrated and googled "How long does it take meditation to work?" When there was no definitive answer, I threw my hands up and said, "See, this is why I have to make pies!"

I saw Dr. Huh weekly, then monthly, and now only when the need arises, like when I get anxious about the holidays or I have work-related FOMO (fear of missing out). Talk therapy—"What happened? Why am I this way?"—helped immensely when sadness and despair tainted every experience I had and I just wanted to rake my jagged feelings over the coals till they were ground down into pebbles. When I felt stronger, I tried cognitive behavioural therapy—"Time is money: stop your whining and set some goals." The part of CBT I like best is identifying behaviours that have worked well in the past, then repeating them.

What's the last time that I remember feeling energized and optimistic?

Playing Beyoncé when I jog so I can pretend to be one of her backup dancers.

Your Answer: _____

_____

When is the last time I remember feeling carefree, in my full dingbat glory?

Chilling with my closest friends.

Your Answer: _____

_____

When is the last time I remember feeling mentally engaged?
Listening to a Malcolm Gladwell audiobook.

Your Answer: _____

_____

While I'm not successful at channelling feelings of happiness out of thin air, I can do the things that make me optimistic, carefree, and engaged. Between these healthful activities and avoiding my triggers (comparing myself to others, going broke trying to duplicate Lady Gaga's wardrobe, watching the Daytime Emmys), I felt more in charge than usual. And just like pulling the cord on a motorboat sometimes takes twenty sputtering tries while you're thinking, "Hurry up and catch, motor, so that I'm not stuck here in the middle of the lake with Randy peeing overboard" before it finally starts and the motor hums loudly to signal you're ready to go, I had to try new approaches over and over until, months in, I realized, "Hey, I'm down to two hours of TV per day, and I haven't felt like the cat's a better person than me in weeks!"

Striving for these small, achievable goals every day has given me a rich life in a different kind of way. "Managing it" is not too shabby. I was never much into lofty New Year's goals anyway; in January, gyms are full, and by March, they're empty (so I've heard? I don't really go to gyms, not even yoga class).

PAT: But you just said you ran into that guy at yoga.
ME: Yeah, 'cause his yoga class is next to my pedi place.
PAT: Oh.

Watching for signs of depression is a lifelong commitment because I'm considered "in remission," not cured. I still feel traces of weakness, because I didn't get a full lobotomy. When I hit a setback (because my insomnia's back or I'm "just not up for this sh*t today" or the house is one-dead-chicken-under-a-filing-cabinet away from being on an episode of *Hoarders*), I might land back on the blue sofa, where I pity myself for hours and binge-watch reality shows and dip bananas straight into the peanut butter jar like it is Fun Dip 'cause getting a spoon is too much work. Then I'll wake up the next day and be anchored again to my simple goals that keep me on the straight and narrow:

- write for two hours
- jog the dog
- make the kids laugh
- go to bed at a decent hour, eat at regular intervals, get some sunshine (basically, live the dream life of a senior citizen)
- fill out kids' school forms so this time I'm the second last, and not last, parent to hand them in

Ya just keep on truckin'. When I fall below a 7/10 for more than a few days, I check in with my mom or Scott or my psychiatrist. I will gladly return to weekly therapy and medication if and when I need it.

PAT: You're not taking anything?

ME: Oh, uh, no. Although I wouldn't recommend anyone stop taking medication without a hearty "You go, girl!" from their doctor, we made a plan for me to wean off of them two years ago. And yes, I hear you, naysayers.

PAT: I didn't say anything!

ME: Someone somewhere did, because there are loud arguments for and against antidepressants. But I am not suggesting anything, and I am not *not* suggesting anything. Just sharing *my* experience. I know nothing. I repeat: nothing.

PAT: Oh, 'cause I was going to stop taking my prescription today just based on your book.

ME: What? Pat, wait! Talk to your d—

PAT: Kidding, kidding.

ME: Heh-heh, you had me there. Good one!

Coming off medication turned me back into a toddler who doesn't know how to properly channel their emotions. Where I was once slightly measured, I was now doing an impression of all three bears from Goldilocks, puffing up brazenly over a $2 carnival prize, or sentimentally over-sharing with an uninterested cashier. I was painting with a palette of twenty-four instead of twelve, and these new colours had me happy-crying again for the first time in years—set off by a church notice board or saccharine holiday commercials or my kids saying "thank you" instead of "seriously?" when I put steamed veggies on the table. And I happy-cry at marathons again, too; awed by the runners' drive to meet the challenge. And now when I think about it, I wonder how many people are running their own marathons every single day: being a single parent, dealing with an invisible illness, juggling a marriage *and* an affair (I'm assuming it's harder than it looks), managing to stay in the race despite it all.

My marathon is putting my mental health above all else. I've lost a few gigs because I won't do overnight shoots or I'm too much of a loner to commit to a creative partner or I'm uncomfortable networking at bars, but new opportunities have filled in those gaps. While I can't help anyone on an individual level (within two days of helping a friend through her breakdown, I was back on the sofa), as a speaker I'm often invited to be a human loudspeaker for those stuck in a negative space. At a recent fundraiser for mental health, I had the pleasure of introducing an inspiring young woman named Jillian who had suffered from debilitating depression and anxiety as a teenager. After she shared her story with eloquence and self-compassion, I asked the audience to let her know "we have your back" and they broke into a loud, encouraging cheer.

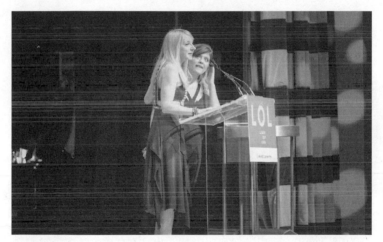

With Jillian Duffy at the George Hull Centre for Children and Families 2017 Laugh Out Loud Fundraiser. Photo courtesy of Kevin Pollock.

We may have been suffering in silence up until recent years, but there's an army, a community of support building. We'll keep yammering away until dealing with mental health is as stigma-free as brushing your teeth or applying sunscreen—just a normal part of our upkeep.

I was recently at a party where someone asked about a talk I had given on depression. She was very beautiful and had clothing that didn't have pet hair all over it and her lipstick hadn't rubbed off on her teeth so I basically thought she was amazing. She tilted her head to the side and said, "You know, I see the news, and all the suffering in the world, and I just can't imagine letting the small stuff get me down." I had heard this before, in many variations—

"Don't you see how good you have it?"
"Mind over matter, right?"
"You don't see me crying about that"

—all implying that depression is a hobby for lazy whiners. And since I had about as much self-esteem as a potato, I used to silently wince at those remarks. This time I carefully replied, "Yeah, I'm not sure that being depressed is caused by a narrow perspective, or a lack of appreciation, because it's an actual illness. I mean, I've never met someone with type 2 diabetes and thought, 'See, I've always just eaten bags of delicious sugar and been fine, so I'm not sure why you can't figure it out.' A gentler thing to say when you hear someone is depressed is 'Sorry, that must be difficult' or some variation on that—well, I suppose you could lose the 'sorry' if you're not Canadian—but I'm just saying is all!" Not quite a mic-drop moment because she then asked, "Are you ok? You're sweaty and red all of a sudden," but I will squeak it from the mountaintop like a proud Swiss horn player every chance I get:

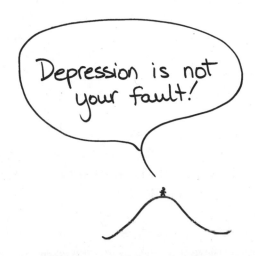

So many people are supporting the cause: for some people it's being a good listener, for others it's tweeting out a message of support or fundraising, and for others it's just trying to get out of bed. And even those people, all by themselves, are part of this army. I hope they know there is strength rallying behind them.

So there ya go. That's it. The end.

PAT: Wait. That's it? What about Scott?

ME: Oh right. Crap. Sorry, Scott.

SCOTT: You make up for it in other ways.

ME: I do!

SCOTT: And by the way, can we talk about some of this stuff you're sharing about us, 'cause I didn't consent to any—

ME: Shhh shhh shhh. Don't worry, Scott. I'll explain it all later.

SCOTT: But I—

Anyway, I am a handful and he is tolerant and that makes for many adventures, which is exactly what we signed up for in the first place. I feel so much gratitude to Scott, and I guess to us, as a couple, for sticking it out. A year and change after I was diagnosed, I proposed to Scott all over again, and we went to Mexico with friends to renew our vows. Of course I didn't want to pay for a whole rental, so I acted as minister AND bride, we used the gazebo that was set up for a wedding later in the day, brought flowers from our room as bouquets, and gladly accepted my daughter's offer to show us a made-up dance as the entertainment. The event concluded with me yelling, "Scatter! The real wedding party's coming!"

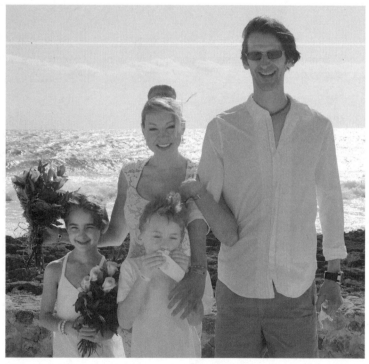

When you ask some passerby in a thong to be your photographer, you're not guaranteed to get the whole wedding party looking toward the camera.

On a trip to that same resort two years later, Genna, feeling self-conscious about her lack of recommitment, decided on the spot that she and Anson would renew their *vowels*, and proceeded to slowly repeat "a-e-i-o-u and sometimes y" while looking into each other's eyes. Genius.

Sometimes I see all the beauty and friendship around me and I'll shake my head, dumbfounded that I am susceptible to depression. I'll wish I could have a do-over of my kids' early years. I'll wish I'd made more of my early career, or that I'd gotten help sooner or not been so desperate to feel beautiful that I got my hair cut in a bob (when your face is round and your neck's a pencil, a bob makes it looks like you're doing a full-time impression of a lollipop). I asked my "1-2-3" grandmother what I could do to get over regret, and she got a twisted look on her face like I'd just asked what I could do to get over blinking. "Well, everyone has regrets. Every single person. Try your best and when you make a mistake, forgive yourself. Then pick yourself up because there's work to be done." Her voice has joined Little Laura and Little Randy over my shoulders and pushes me forward.

I will always see the door in the corner that leads to depression, because it will always be there. But it's just a door and I'm making joyful sport of avoiding it. Maybe our whole lives will be spent trying, channelling all the tenacity that's in us to keep looking for a clear path. How beautiful would that be, to discover we are the most optimistic of them all.

Would you look at that? I'm all out of sour grapes. Just room for butter tarts now. And pie. Oooh, pie. I've gotta go. That store-bought pie shell's not gonna leap into a glass pan so it can pretend it's homemade all by itself.

ME: Oh, and Pat?

PAT: Yes?

ME: I don't really know you. But just wanted to say that I really appreciate that you made it through the book. Thanks for sticking around.

PAT: Oh. Sure.

ME: I think that anyone with enough compassion to read about someone else's journey must be pretty terrific. Take care.

PAT: You, too.

ME: Thanks. Bye.

PAT: Bye.

ME: ... are you still there?

PAT: Yes.

ME: Ok, signing off now. Close the book so I can go.

PAT: Ok.

(*PAUSE*)

ME: Have you closed the book?

PAT: Well, no, 'cause you're still writing.

ME: Ok, ok, I'm stopping.

PAT: Closing the book.

ME: Turning off the computer.

ME AND PAT: Bye!

Acknowledgments

· · · · · ·

THIS WAS A difficult book to get published. "Dig deeper," they said, even after I explained that when the going gets tough, some of us need a frolic in the shallows. When I needed encouragement, Adrean Turner, Amy Moore-Benson, and Farah Perelmuter cheered me on. Laura Cain, Jennifer Gillespie, Genna duPlessis, Kelly Smith, Lisa Gilroy, Ian Sirota, and George Holmes gave me thoughtful and supportive feedback. Scott McCrickard brainstormed with me. Mike MacDonald generously met with me to discuss depression and comedy. Simon B. Cotter, Jennifer Irwin, James Cunningham, and Dean Young shared their anecdotes for the Humiliation Fee chapter. Aisha Alfa, Kathryn Greenwood, and Dr. Shimi Kang read my material and provided thoughtful quotes for the book's cover. Don Ferguson allowed me to borrow an *Air Farce* promo pic for the book's cover, and Rodney Daw took said pic. Grand Wave Entertainment and Speakers' Spotlight propelled me forward. And my Junction Moms' group always reminds me that we've got each other's backs, unconditionally. Thanks, guys.

Stephanie Fysh was the greatest editor I could hope for, and the whole team at Page Two Strategies helped turn this dream into a reality. Thanks for signing me up, Jessica Finkelstein; for enthusiastically keeping me on track, Trena White and Gabrielle Narsted; for designing this classy book, Peter Cocking; and for using your copy-editing skills to stop me from embarrassing myself, Erin Parker.

I've gotta thank Scott for allowing me to splash our private business all over these pages for the greater good. Yup, he really is that nice a guy. My big-hearted kids gave me permission to write about this important subject even though it might lead to some weird questions in the schoolyard. Alexa and Jordan, even if you didn't understand, you said yes for the benefit of others. Thanks for being generous. Thank you, Grampa "Poopa," for teaching me to laugh it off, and thank you, Nan "Noon," for your wisdom. To my parents, for always having good advice, and for being a soft place to land when I don't take that advice. To all my relatives, for your sense of humour. You're my backbone.

Thank you all so much.

In all seriousness...

Some Resources

· · · · ·

WELL, PAT, TOMFOOLERY and shenanigans aside, if you're going through a rough time, I hope you know that there are always people available to help. If you feel you need support, please *talk to someone*. That may be

- your doctor
- a crisis phone line: www.yourlifecounts.org/need-help/ crisis-lines
- an online crisis line: www.imalive.org

And if you want to understand more, or get involved, here are some great places to start:

- Healthy Minds Canada: https://healthymindscanada.ca
- The George Hull Centre for Children and Families: www.georgehullcentre.on.ca
- Anxiety and Depression Association of America: https://adaa.org

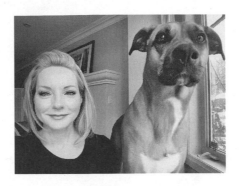

About the Author

* * * * *

JESSICA HOLMES IS a Canadian comedian, actress, and improviser best known for her work on the *Royal Canadian Air Farce* and *The Holmes Show*. As a stand-up, she has opened for comedians Jerry Seinfeld, Ellen DeGeneres, and Russell Peters, as well as icons like Oprah Winfrey and Deepak Chopra. She's performed with The Second City and Just for Laughs, and she's appeared on the TV shows *Little Big Kid, The Itch,* and *Wild Card*. Her first memoir, *I Love Your Laugh: Finding the Light in My Screwball Life,* was published by McClelland & Stewart in 2011. After battling postpartum depression and "regular, run-of-the-mill, garden-variety depression" (her words), Holmes began openly sharing her mental health story using humour. She is the daughter of a Mormon father and a feminist mother (yes, that should be a sitcom), and she lives in Toronto with her husband and two kids.